بسم الله الرحمن الرحيم

ABOUT THE AUTHOR

Under the pen-name HARUN YAHYA, the author has published many books on political and faith-related issues. An important body of his work deals with the materialistic world view and the impact of it in world history and politics. (The pen-name is formed from the names 'Harun' [Aaron] and 'Yahya' [John] in the esteemed memory of the two Prophets who struggled against infidelity.)

His works include The 'Secret Hand' in Bosnia, The Holocaust Hoax, Behind the Scenes of Terrorism, Israel's Kurdish Card, A National Strategy for Turkey, Solution: The Morals of the Qur'an, Darwin's Antagonism Against the Turks, The Calamities Darwinism Caused Humanity, The Evolution Deceit, Perished Nations, The Golden Age, Allah's Artistry in Colour, Glory is Everywhere, The Truth of the Life of This World, Confessions of Evolutionists, The Blunders of Evolutionists, The Dark Magic of Darwinism, The Religion of Darwinism, The Qur'an Leads the Way to Science, The Real Origin of Life, The Creation of the Universe, Miracles of the Qur'an, The Design in Nature, Self-Sacrifice and Intelligent Behaviour Models in Animals, Eternity Has Already Begun, Children Darwin Was Lying!, The End of Darwinism, Deep Thinking, Timelessness and the Reality of Fate, Never Plead Ignorance, The Secrets of DNA, The Miracle of the Atom, The Miracle in the Cell, The Miracle of the Immune System, The Miracle in the Eye, The Creation Miracle in Plants, The Miracle in the Spider, The Miracle in the Ant, The Miracle in the Gnat, The Miracle in the Honeybee, The Miracle of Seed, The Miracle in the Termite.

Among his booklets are The Mystery of the Atom, The Collapse of the Theory of Evolution: The Fact of Creation, The Collapse of Materialism, The End of Materialism, The Blunders of Evolutionists 1, The Blunders of Evolutionists 2, The Microbiological Collapse of Evolution, The Fact of Creation, The Collapse of the Theory of Evolution in 20 Questions, The Biggest Deception in the History of Biology: Darwinism.

The author's other works on Quranic topics include: Ever Thought About the Truth?, Devoted to Allah, Abandoning the Society of Ignorance, Paradise, The Theory of Evolution, The Moral Values of the Qur'an, Knowledge of the Qur'an, Qur'an Index, Emigrating for the Cause of Allah, The Character of Hypocrites in the Qur'an, The Secrets of the Hypocrite, The Names of Allah, Communicating the Message and Disputing in the Qur'an, The Basic Concepts in the Qur'an, Answers from the Qur'an, Death Resurrection Hell, The Struggle of the Messengers, The Avowed Enemy of Man: Satan, Idolatry, The Religion of the Ignorant, The Arrogance of Satan, Prayer in the Qur'an, The Importance of Conscience in the Qur'an, The Day of Resurrection, Never Forget, Disregarded Judgements of the Qur'an, Human Characters in the Society of Ignorance, The Importance of Patience in the Qur'an, General Information from the Qur'an, Quick Grasp of Faith 1-2-3, The Crude Reasoning of Disbelief, The Mature Faith, Before You Regret, Our Messengers Say, The Mercy of Believers, The Fear of Allah, The Nightmare of Disbelief, Prophet Isa Will Come, Beauties Presented by the Qur'an for Life, Bouquet of the Beauties of Allah 1-2-3-4, The Iniquity Called "Mockery", The Secret of the Test, The True Wisdom According to the Qur'an, The Struggle with the Religion of Irreligion, The School of Yusuf, The Alliance of the Good, Slanders Spread Against Muslims Throughout History, The Importance of Following the Good Word, Why Do You Deceive Yourself?, Islam: The Religion of Ease, Enthusiasm and Vigor in the Qur'an, Seeing Good in Everything, How does the Unwise Interpret the Qur'an?, Some Secrets of the Qur'an, The Courage of Believers.

THE
MIRACLE
OF THE
IMMUNE SYSTEM

First published 2001
© Goodword Books 2003
Reprinted 2002, 2003

ISBN 81-87570-83-0

Goodword Books Pvt. Ltd.
1, Nizamuddin West Market
New Delhi 110 013
Tel. 435 5454, 435 6666
Fax 435 7333, 435 7980
e-mail: info@goodwordbooks.com

THE
MIRACLE
OF THE
IMMUNE SYSTEM

HARUN YAHYA

Goodword

TO THE READER

The reason why a special chapter is assigned to the collapse of the theory of evolution is that this theory constitutes the basis of all anti-spiritual philosophies. Since Darwinism rejects the fact of creation, and therefore the existence of Allah, during the last 140 years it has caused many people to abandon their faith or fall into doubt. Therefore, showing that this theory is a deception is a very important duty, which is strongly related to the religion. It is imperative that this important service be rendered to everyone. Some of our readers may find the chance to read only one of our books. Therefore, we think it appropriate to spare a chapter for a summary of this subject.

In all the books by the author, faith-related issues are explained in the light of the Qur'anic verses and people are invited to learn Allah's words and to live by them. All the subjects that concern Allah's verses are explained in such a way as to leave no room for doubt or question marks in the reader's mind. The sincere, plain and fluent style employed ensures that everyone of every age and from every social group can easily understand the books. This effective and lucid narrative makes it possible to read them in a single sitting. Even those who rigorously reject spirituality are influenced by the facts recounted in these books and cannot refute the truthfulness of their contents.

This book and all the other works of the author can be read individually or discussed in a group at a time of conversation. Those readers who are willing to profit from the books will find discussion very useful in the sense that they will be able to relate their own reflections and experiences to one another.

In addition, it will be a great service to the religion to contribute to the presentation and reading of these books, which are written solely for the good pleasure of Allah. All the books of the author are extremely convincing. For this reason, for those who want to communicate the religion to other people, one of the most effective methods is to encourage them to read these books.

It is hoped that the reader will take time to look through the review of other books on the final pages of the book, and appreciate the rich source of material on faith-related issues, which are very useful and a pleasure to read.

In these books, you will not find, as in some other books, the personal views of the author, explanations based on dubious sources, styles that are unobservant of the respect and reverence due to sacred subjects, nor hopeless, doubt-creating, and pessimistic accounts that create deviations in the heart.

CONTENTS

PREFACE

One the most important factors for the continued existence of any country is its defence capability. As a nation, it must be in a constant state of preparedness to face all kinds of threats and dangers from external and internal sources. No matter how well developed and advanced a country may be, if it fails to defend itself, it could be brought to ruin with the launching of even a minor military offensive against it, or even a well-directed and unanticipated terrorist act. In the face of such threats, neither its natural resources, its technological prowess, not its economy will be of any avail. If the country in question is unable to defend itself, it may even cease to exist.

This is one of the reasons why significant amounts of the national income is regularly allocated to defence; nowadays, armed forces have to be provided with the most advanced weaponry, tools and equipment fitted with the latest technological features, and meticulous training has to be given to soldiers in an all-out attempt to keep defence systems fully functional.

No less than countries, people too have to be concerned about their defence, if they want to lead a healthy and peaceful life. They inevitably have to protect themselves and their possession against criminal acts, such as theft and murder, as well as against natural disasters, such as accidents, fire, earthquakes and floods.

But this is not the end of the matter. Human beings have other enemies, which go unseen by them and, as such, are often ignored. Actually, these enemies are much more resilient than the others. Serious measures must, therefore, be taken to guard against them.

Who, or what then these enemies that keep human beings under constant threat?

They are bacteria, viruses, and similar microscopic organisms, which may exist in the water we drink, the food we eat, the house we live in, and the office where we work. In essence, they are everywhere.

Most interestingly, in spite of being surrounded by such a serious threat, we make no effort whatsoever to protect ourselves against it. This is because there is a mechanism within our bodies, which undertakes this task on our behalf, providing the necessary protection for us, without causing us the slightest disturbance. This is "The Defence System".

It is one of the most important and amazing systems operating within our bodies, for it undertakes one of the most vital missions of life. We may not be aware of it, but all the elements of the immune system protect our bodies just like the soldiers of a huge army. The defence cells that protect the human body against invaders, such as bacteria, viruses, and similar micro-organisms, are equipped with extraordinary abilities. The patterns of intelligence, effort, and sacrifice, which these cells display during the war they wage in the body, astonish everyone who learns about them.

People in general would like to know what makes them ill, how illnesses take complete control of their bodies, what causes fever, fatigue, pain in their bones and joints, and which processes take place in their bodies throughout their illnesses.

The main purpose of this book is to explore how this system, which protects the human body just like a disciplined, organized army, has come into being and how it works.

These two points will lead us to very important conclusions. First, we shall together witness the uniqueness and the perfection in Allah's creation. Second, we shall observe what contradictions the theory of evolution, a superstitious belief having no verification whatsoever, includes within its own reasoning, and on what an unsound basis it was erected.

Before proceeding to the main topic, it will be useful to state another important point: In books on the immune system, you will often see statements such as:

"We do not yet know how this formed..."

"The reason still remains unknown..."

"Research on the topic is under way ..."

"According to a theory..."

These statements are actually important confessions. These are expressions of the helplessness people experience at the outset of the 21st century — even with all the latest technology and accumulated knowledge at their disposal — in the face of the miraculous work these tiny cells accomplish. The tasks achieved by these microorganisms include such intricate operations that the human mind can barely grasp the details of this well established system. There is obviously a secret wisdom hidden in the immune system which eludes man's understanding.

As you read this book, you will witness the superiority of this wisdom, hidden both in your cells and in other details pertaining to your body. The ultimate conclusion is that this could only be the wisdom of a supreme "Creator".

Science may one day succeed in solving all the secrets of the immune system and even produce a similar artificial system by imitating the actions of these cells. No doubt, this task will require highly educated professionals using the most sophisticated technology and instruments available, working in highly advanced laboratories. The most important point here is that the accomplishment of such a task would once again invalidate the theory of evolution, proving that such a system cannot originate by coincidence.

The likelihood of the spontaneous development of a mechanism such as the defence system currently seems too remote. As scientists unravel the secrets of this system, they are enthralled by the design they encounter. The points that are revealed lead to many other questions, which make the wisdom and consciousness in the cell all the more apparent. Therefore, it has become very clear that the defence system, like all the other systems in the body, could not have developed gradually, just by chance, as suggested by the theory of evolution.

The main purpose of this book is to introduce you to these "brave warriors" within you, while also proving to you that this mind-boggling system is a special sign of creation. In relation to this, we will see how the scenarios formulated by the theory of evolution are demolished and rendered meaningless when faced with the facts. The topic which will be particularly highlighted here, is not the biological details of the defence system, which are easily accessible in any book of biology or medicine, but the miraculous aspect of the system. We have especially avoided the unnecessary use of biological and physiological terms in order to make the contents of the book easily understandable to readers of all ages and professions.

Lastly, we want to remind you that even now, you are totally indebted to your defence system if you are able to read this book peacefully, without being infected by the microbes all around you. Had the immune system not existed in your body, you would never have been able to read this book, having left this world even before you learned reading and writing.

INTRODUCTION

Before delving into the astounding details of the war of defence fought in the innermost recesses of our bodies, we must first have a general look at the defence system and its elements.

Briefly, the defence system may be defined as "an extremely disciplined, hard-working and organized army that protects the body from the clutches of external enemies." In this multi-faceted war, the main duty of the elements fighting in the front line is to prevent the enemy cells, such as bacteria or viruses, from entering the body.

Although it is not easy for the enemy organisms to enter the body, they exert themselves to the utmost to reach their ultimate goal of invading the body. When they successfully do so, after overcoming various obstacles such as the skin, and the respiratory and digestive tracts, they will find tough warriors waiting for them. These tough warriors are produced and trained in specialized centres such as the bone marrow, spleen, thymus, and lymph nodes. These warriors are "the defence cells" referred to as the macrophages and lymphocytes.

First, various types of phagocytes, which are called the "the eater cells" will swing into action. Then the macrophages, another specific type of phagocytes, take their turn. They all destroy the enemy by engulfing it. Macrophages also perform other duties such as summoning other defence cells to the battleground, and raising the body temperature. The rise in temperature at the onset of a sickness is very important, for the afflicted the person will feel fatigued by it and need to rest, thus reserving the energy needed to fight against the enemies.

If these elements of the immune system prove insufficient against the enemies penetrating the body, then lymphocytes, the champions of the system, come into play. Lymphocytes are of two types; B cells and T cells. These are again further divided into sub groups.

The helper T cells are next in reaching the battleground after the macrophages. They may be considered the administrative agents of the system. After the helper T cells identify the enemy, they warn other cells in order to initiate a war against it.

Thus alerted, the killer T cells come into play to destroy the besieged enemy.

The B cells are the armaments factory of the human body. Following their stimulation by the helper T cells, they immediately start to produce a sort of weapon called the "antibody".

After the alarm is over, suppressor T cells stop the activity of all defence cells, and therefore prevent the war from lasting any longer than is necessary.

However, the mission of the defence army has not yet ended. The warrior cells, called the memory cells, store necessary information about the enemy in their memories and keep it for years. This will enable the immune system to mount a quick defence against the same enemy at later meetings with it.

There are many more incredible factors hidden in the details of the defence system, which we have very briefly outlined above. As mentioned before, in this book, these extraordinary events are told in an easy-to-understand way.

THE DEFENCE SYSTEM

Around 250 years ago, scientists discovered, after the invention of microscope, that we live together with many tiny creatures, which we cannot see with the naked eye. These creatures are present everywhere — from the air we inhale, to the water we drink, to any object which comes in contact with the surface of our body. It was also discovered that these creatures penetrate the human body.

Although the existence of this enemy was discovered two and a half centuries ago, most of the secrets of the "defence system" that fights a vigorous war against it have not yet been uncovered. This molecular system in the body is activated automatically according to an exquisite plan the minute a stranger makes its way in, declaring an all-out war against it. When we take a quick look at how the system works, we see that every phase takes place according to a meticulous plan.

The System That Never Sleeps

Whether we are aware of it or not, millions of operations and reactions take place in our bodies every second. This action continues even when we are asleep.

This intense activity occurs in periods of time which from our viewpoint are very short. There is a significant difference between the notion of time in our daily lives and the biological time of our body. The span of one second that represents a very short time period in our daily life would pass for a very long time for many working systems and organs in our bodies. If all the activities performed by all the organs, tissues and cells of our body in one second were written down, the result would be so inconceivable as to push the limits of the human mind.

One vital system, which is involved in constant activity, never shirking its duty, is the defence system. This system protects the body from all kinds of invaders day and night and works with great assiduity, just like a fully-equipped army for the host body, which it serves.

Each system, organ, or group of cells within the body represents a whole within a perfect labour distribution. Any defect in the system ruins the order. And the defence system is indispensable.

Would we be able to survive in the absence of the defence system? Or what sort of life would we have if this system failed to fulfill some of its functions?

It is not hard to make a guess. Some examples in the world of medicine make clear how vital the immune system is. The story of a patient cited in many related sources shows how difficult life would be in case of any defect in the defence system.

This patient was placed immediately after his birth in a sterile plastic tent, which nothing was allowed to penetrate. The patient was forbidden to touch any other human being. As he grew up, he was placed in a larger plastic tent. He had to wear a specially designed outfit similar to an astronaut's to get out of this tent. What prevented this patient from living a normal life like other people?

Following his birth, the patient's defence system had not developed normally. There was no army in his body to protect him from the enemies.

The boy's doctors were well aware of what could happen if he entered normal surroundings. He would immediately catch a cold, causing diseases to develop in his throat; he would suffer from one infection after another, despite being given antibiotics and other medical treatments. Before long, medical treatment would lose its effect, resulting in the death of the boy.

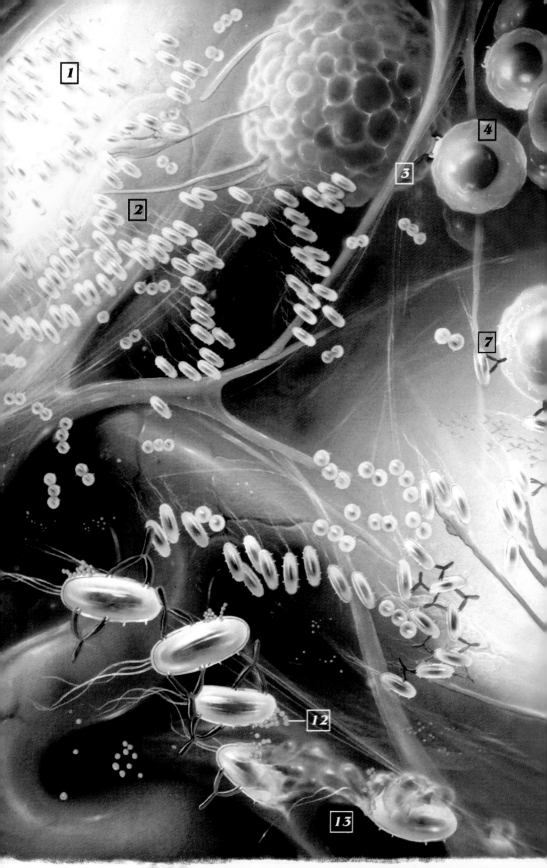

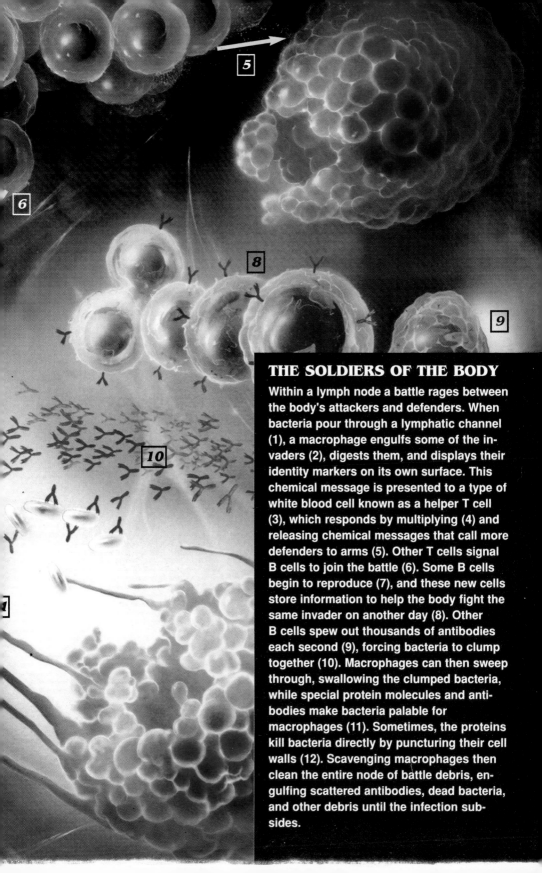

THE SOLDIERS OF THE BODY

Within a lymph node a battle rages between the body's attackers and defenders. When bacteria pour through a lymphatic channel (1), a macrophage engulfs some of the invaders (2), digests them, and displays their identity markers on its own surface. This chemical message is presented to a type of white blood cell known as a helper T cell (3), which responds by multiplying (4) and releasing chemical messages that call more defenders to arms (5). Other T cells signal B cells to join the battle (6). Some B cells begin to reproduce (7), and these new cells store information to help the body fight the same invader on another day (8). Other B cells spew out thousands of antibodies each second (9), forcing bacteria to clump together (10). Macrophages can then sweep through, swallowing the clumped bacteria, while special protein molecules and antibodies make bacteria palable for macrophages (11). Sometimes, the proteins kill bacteria directly by puncturing their cell walls (12). Scavenging macrophages then clean the entire node of battle debris, engulfing scattered antibodies, dead bacteria, and other debris until the infection subsides.

At best, he would be able to live only for a few months or a few years out of this safe environment. So the boy's entire world was forever bounded by the walls of his plastic tent.

After sometime, the doctors and his family placed the boy in a completely germfree room which had been specially prepared in his house. However, all these efforts were useless. In his early teens, when a bone transplant failed. [1]

The boy's family, doctors, the staff of the hospital where he had earlier stayed, and pharmaceutical companies did their best to keep him alive. Although absolutely everything was tried, and the boy's place of residence was continuously disinfected, his death could not be prevented.

This end clearly shows that it is impossible for a human being to sur-

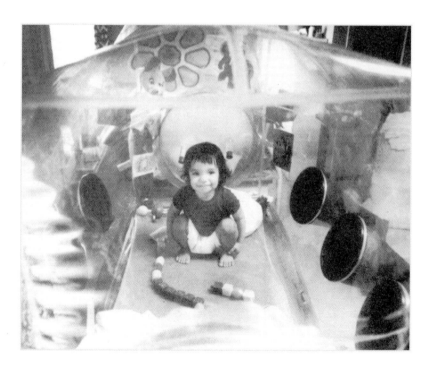

The boy in a bubble. Born in 1971 with no immune defenses, he was delivered in a germfree environment at a hospital but his death could not be prevented.

vive without a defence system to protect him from microbes. This is evidence that the immune system must have existed complete and intact since the advent of the first man. Therefore, it is out of question that such a system could have developed gradually over a long lapse of time as the theory of evolution claims. A human being without a defence system, or with a malfunctioning one, would shortly die as seen in this example.

BESIEGED CASTLE: THE HUMAN BODY

I t is a fact that even though we try to live in clean environments, we share these places with many micro-organisms. If you had the chance to view the room you are currently sitting in with a microscope, you would immediately see the millions of organisms you live with.

In this situation, the individual resembles a "besieged castle". Needless to say, such a castle, which is surrounded by countless enemies, must be protected in a very complete and organized manner. Human beings are created along with this perfect protection they need, and are not, therefore, entirely defenceless against these enemies. The "micro" guards in our bodies never leave us alone and fight for us on many fronts.

The invader cells that want to take control of the body first have to

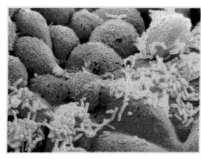

Masses of influenza bacteria on the nasal epithelium.

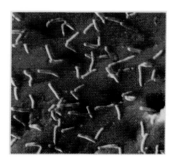

Bacteria on a recently brushed tooth.

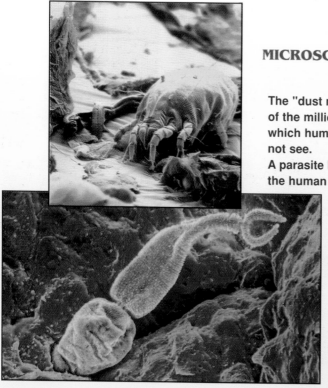

MICROSCOPIC MONSTERS

The "dust mite" (left) is only one of the millions of organisms with which humans live with but cannot see.

A parasite larva while breaching the human skin (bottom). This organism will make its way to the blood stream through the skin, and settle into the vessels to multiply. It uses incredible tactics to escape from the body's army of defence, such as camouflaging itself with the material it rips off from the host cell.

fight their way through the front line of the body. Even though these fronts have their weaknesses at times, the enemy is hardly ever allowed to pass through them. The first front the enemy must penetrate is our skin.

The Protective Armour of Our Body: The Skin

The skin, which covers the entire body of a human being just like a sheath, is full of amazing features. Its ability to repair and renew itself, its non-permeability by water, despite the existence of tiny pores on its surface as opposed to its function of discharging water through perspiration,

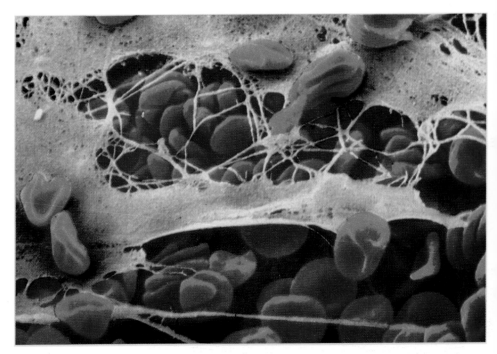

The first defense response of the organism against its dangerous invaders is the rapid self-repairing of the skin tissue following the infliction of a wound. When such a wound ruptures the skin, defence cells immediately travel to the injured area to fight with the foreign cell and to remove the debris of the affected tissue. Later, some other defence cells enhance the production of fibrin, which is a protein that rapidly re-covers the wound with a fibrous network. This picture is of a fibrin that has spread over some red blood cells.

The invader cells that want to take control of the body first have to fight their way through the front line of the body. Even though these fronts have their weaknesses at times, the enemy is hardly ever allowed to pass through them. The first front the enemy must penetrate is our skin.

The Protective Armour of Our Body: The Skin

The skin, which covers the entire body of a human being just like a sheath, is full of amazing features. Its ability to repair and renew itself, its non-permeability by water, despite the existence of tiny pores on its surface as opposed to its function of discharging water through perspiration,

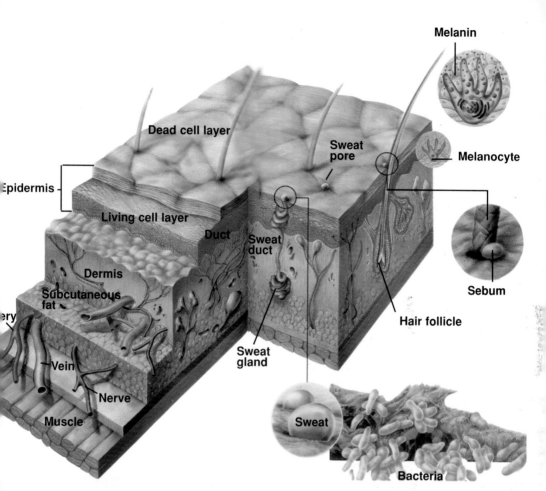

Melanin

Dead cell layer

Sweat pore

Melanocyte

Epidermis

Living cell layer

Duct

Sweat duct

Dermis

Subcutaneous fat

Sebum

ery

Vein

Hair follicle

Nerve

Sweat gland

Muscle

Sweat

Bacteria

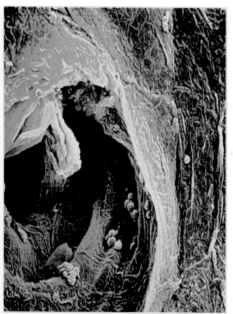

AN IN-DEPTH VIEW OF THE SKIN

Above is a cross-section of the skin. The sweat droplets secreted from the skin play a variety of roles in the body. In addition bringing down the body temperature, they provide nutrition for certain bacteria and fungi living on the surface of the skin, and produce acidic waste materials such as lactic acid which helps decrease the PH level of the skin. This acidic medium on the skin surface creates a hostile environment for any harmful bacteria that are looking for a place to live.

At the left is a close-up of the sweat gland entrance. Here, too, you will find bacteria just like everywhere else on the skin.

its extremely flexible structure, allowing free movement, as opposed to its being thick enough to avoid easy rupture, its ability to protect the body from the heat, the cold, and harmful sunrays are only a few of the features of the skin that have been specially created for human beings. Here, we will deal with a particular feature of this extraordinary wrapping paper: its ability to protect the body from disease-causing micro-organisms. If the body is considered a castle besieged by enemies, we can safely refer to the skin as the strong walls of this castle.

The main protective function of the skin is realized via the dead cell layers constituting the outer section of the skin. Each new cell produced by cell division moves from the inner section of the skin towards the surface. While doing this, the liquid element (cytoplasm) of the cell interior transforms into a resistant protein known as keratin. During the process, the cell dies. The newly formed keratin substance has a very hard structure and is not therefore subject to decomposition by digestive enzymes, which is a sign of its resistance. Thus, invaders such as bacteria and fungi will be unable to find anything to rip off from the outer layer of the

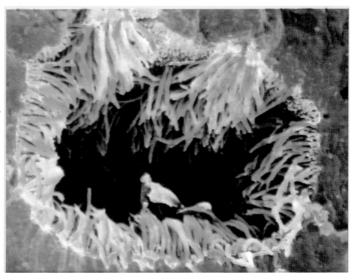

This picture, which is magnified 5900 times, shows the cells in the trachea (blue). They use their glands (yellow) to secrete a substance that traps the particles in the air.

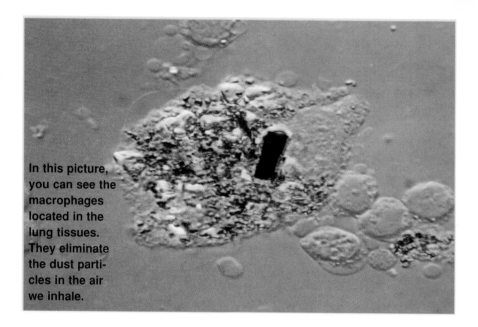

In this picture, you can see the macrophages located in the lung tissues. They eliminate the dust particles in the air we inhale.

skin.

Moreover, dead outer cells containing keratin are constantly shed from the skin surface. The new cells that come from beneath to replace the discarded ones form an impenetrable barrier in that area.

The organisms on the skin fulfill another protective function of the skin. A group of harmless microbes live on the skin, which have adapted to its acidic medium. Feeding on the leftovers stuck on the keratin of the skin, these microbes attack all kinds of foreign bodies to protect their feeding site. The skin, as the host of these microbes, is like a supplementary force that provides external support to the army within the human body.

Protection in Respiration

One of the courses our enemies take to enter our body is the respiratory tract. Hundreds of varied microbes, which are present in the air we inhale, try to gain entry to the body through these passages. However, they are unaware of the barrier set up against them in the nose.

A special secretion in the nasal mucous retains and sweeps out about 80-90% of the micro-organisms that gain entry to the respiratory system directly or through dust particles or other substances.

In addition, the tiny hairlike structures (cilia) on the surface of the cells of the respiratory tract beat upward, causing a current that carries foreign particles to the throat where they are swallowed and disposed of by acid in the stomach. The coughing reflex and sneezing facilitate this function.

The microbes that are able to surmount these barriers and reach the alveoli (lung, bronchus and gingiva) will be ingested by phagocytes. After this phase, phagocytes become mobile and drift upwards with the microbes they have ingested to be finally discharged from the body in different ways.

Each time you breathe, as you are doing now, a war is fought at the border gates of your body of which you are completely unaware. The guards at these border gates fight with the enemy to the death to protect your health.

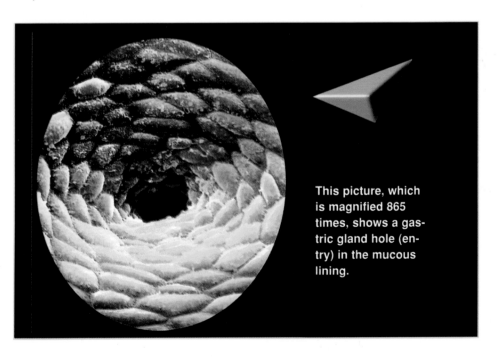

This picture, which is magnified 865 times, shows a gastric gland hole (entry) in the mucous lining.

Protection in the Digestive System

Another vehicle by which microbes gain entry to our body is our food. However, the guards of our body, which are aware of this method used by the microbes, await them in the region where the food finally ends up, which is the stomach. They also have a surprise for the arriving microbes, which is the gastric acid. This acid is quite an unpleasant surprise for the microbes which have overcome all obstacles and reached the stomach. The majority, if not all, of the microbes are defeated by this acid.

Some microbes may overcome this obstacle because they have not made enough contact with the gastric acid, or they have showed resistance. However, these microbes are again subjected to further conflicts with other guards situated on their way. Now, another surprise is at hand for them: the digestive enzymes produced in the small intestine. This time, they cannot get away as easily.

As we have seen, the human body has specially created guards, which protect the human body in every phase of the microbes' assaults.

There are now some important questions raised by this examination.

Who established that microbes living outside would try to penetrate our body through foods, which route the food would follow, how microbes would be destroyed in their final destination, where they would go if they overcame this obstacle, and how in that case they should be exposed to stronger measures? Is it the body cells, which have never been out of the body, and therefore, have no chance of examining the chemical make-up of the microbes outside, and which, moreover, have not received any training in chemistry?

Definitely not. Only Allah, Who created both the external world, and the food in this world, and the body that needs these foods, and the system to digest these foods, is able to create such a defence system.

Another Method: Destroying the Enemy by Another Enemy

There are many other micro-organisms that live within the human body which cause us no harm. What are these organisms that continue with their own life without doing us any harm, and what is their purpose in living within our body?

These groups of micro-organisms, which are gathered in certain parts of the body, are called the normal microbial flora of the body. They do no damage and even have some benefits for the human body.

These micro-organisms provide external support for the defence army against microbes. They benefit the body by preventing foreign microbes from settling in it, because the entry of any microbe into the body is a threat to their own housing site. Since they do not want to be displaced by the invaders, they fight a fierce battle against them. We can think of these micro-organisms as "professional soldiers" fighting for the body. They try to protect the site they live in for their own benefit. In so

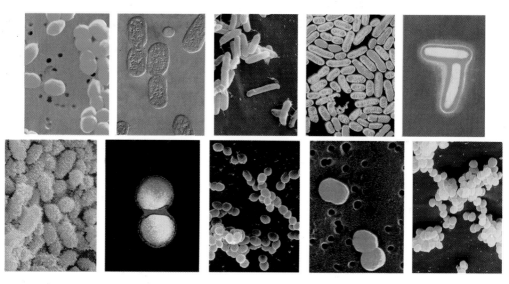

There are hundreds of bacteria in the world. In the above picture, you can see only a few of them.

doing, they complement the fully equipped army in our body.

How do these "professional soldiers" settle in our bodies?

The human embryo has met no enemy during the gestation period in the mother's womb. Following the birth of the child, it makes contact with the environment, and numerous microbes are introduced to the child through the intake of food and by way of the respiratory tract. Some of these microbes die right away, while others are discharged before having the chance to settle down in the body. Some, however, settle in various parts of the body such as the skin, skin ridges, mouth, nose, eyes, upper respiratory tract, digestive tract, and genital organs. These microbes form permanent colonies at these locations and constitute the microbial flora of the human body.

Who are Our Micro Enemies?

Our micro enemies, on the other hand, are micro-organisms, which are not a part of our bodies, yet which have somehow penetrated our bodies, eventually stimulating the defence army therein.

Every foreign cell that enters the body is not, however treated as an enemy. Foreign matter constantly enters our bodies as we eat, drink

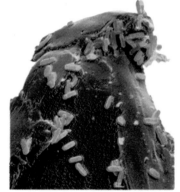

The magnified view of bacteria on the tip of a needle.

water, or take medicine. Yet our body does not initiate a war with it. In order for the defence cells to perceive a foreign substance as an enemy, certain conditions are taken into consideration such as the size of the molecule, its rate of elimination from the body, and its way of entering the body.

Bacteria

Among our innumerable micro enemies, bacteria have an established reputation.

Bacteria, which enter the human body in multiple ways, instigate a fierce war in the body. Sometimes ending up with quite serious illnesses, these wars explicitly reveal the power and ability hidden in an organism the size of a few microns (a micron is one thousandth of a millimeter). Recent research has shown that bacteria have an extraordinary resistance even to the most severe and harsh conditions. Particularly, the bacteria known as spores are resistant to extremely high temperatures and drought for extended periods. This is why it is difficult to destroy certain microbes.

Viruses

The human body resembles a very valuable diamond stored in a safe, receiving the most intensive care and protection. Some of the organisms that try to invade the body act like experienced thieves. One of the best known and most important of these thieves is the virus.

This organism, whose existence we became aware of with the invention of the electron microscope, is too simple-structured and small to be considered even as a cell. Viruses, which vary in sizes ranging from 0.1 to 0.280 microns, are excluded from the world of living things for this reason.[2]

Although categorized as being apart from the world of living beings, viruses indisputably possess at least as exceptional abilities as all other living beings do. A closer examination of the lives of viruses will make this fact more apparent. Viruses

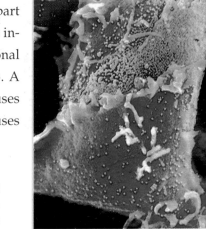

A virus modifying its structure so that it is not identified by the immune system. (The rhinovirus 14)

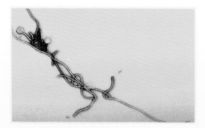

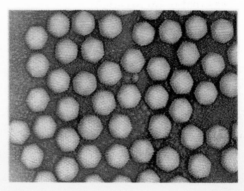

Ebola virus (top left) Influenza virus (bottom left) Common cold virus (bottom right)

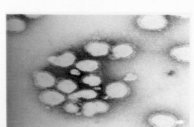

are the compulsory parasites of living beings. This means, they cannot survive if they do not settle into a plant, animal, or human cell, and consume its food and energy. Viruses do not have a system that would enable them to survive on their own. As if they are aware of this, they deftly slip into a cell, and after invading the cell, with the same deftness turn the cell into a "virus production factory" that produces its own copies.

This plan developed by the virus to invade the cell is extremely sophisticated and intelligent. In the first place, the virus must determine whether the cell is appropriate for itself or not. It has to be very careful and meticulous in this decision, for the smallest mistake may cause its death. To avoid such an end, it uses its special receptors to check whether the cell is appropriate for it or not. The next important thing it does is to carefully locate itself within the cell.

The virus confuses the cell with the tactics it employs and avoids observation.

This is how the events develop: the cell transports the new DNA of the virus into its nucleus. Thinking that it produces protein, the cell starts to replicate this new DNA. The DNA of the virus hides itself so furtively that the cell involuntarily becomes the production factory of its own ene-my and produces the very viruses that will eventually destroy it. It is in-deed very difficult for the cell to identify the hereditary make-up of the vi-rus as that of an invader.

The virus locates itself within the cell so well that it almost becomes a part of it. After the multiplication process is over, the virus and other new viruses depart from the cell to repeat the same process in other cells. During the process, depending on the type of the virus and the cell, the virus can kill the host cell, cause harm to it, modify it, or simply do noth-ing.

The question of how the cell, which operates under a very strictly monitored control mechanism, can be deceived into becoming a virus fac-tory is still unanswered. It is quite intriguing that viruses, which have a highly specialized structure, but which are not even classified as living beings, could act so intelligently, think up, and plan such effective strate-gies. The secret of this phenomenon lies in the existence of a Creator, Who created these organisms with the abilities they possess.

The features of the virus are perfectly designed to enable it to make use of the system operating in the cell. It is obvious that the power that created the virus is also well informed about the extremely complex working principles of the cell. This power belongs to Allah, Who created the virus and the cell into which it will settle, as He created the entire uni-verse.

The virus, which, with its miniscule structure, can inflict and some-times even cause the death of the human body, which is millions of times bigger than itself in size, is a being specially created by Allah to remind people of their weaknesses.

INTELLIGENT WEAPONS: THE ANTIBODIES

Antibodies are protein-structured weapons, which are manufactured to fight against the foreign cells entering the human body. These weapons are produced by the B cells, a class of warriors of the immune system.

Antibodies destroy invaders. They have two main functions: The first is to bind to the invader cell, which is the antigen. The second is to decompose the biological structure of the antigen and destroy it.

Swimming in the blood and non-cellular fluid, antibodies bind to disease-causing bacteria and viruses. They mark the foreign molecules to which they bind, so that the body's fighter cells can distinguish them. This way, they also inactivate them. This resembles a tank becoming useless and unable to move or fire shells when it is hit by a guided missile in the battleground. An antibody fits the enemy (antigen) perfectly, just like a key and a lock assembling in a three-dimensional structure.

The human body can produce a compatible antibody for almost every enemy it encounters. Antibodies are not of one type only. According to the structure of every enemy, a specific antibody powerful enough to deal with it is produced. This is because an antibody produced for one disease may not be effective on another.

Manufacturing a specific antibody for each enemy is rather an unusual process, which deserves closer attention. This process can be realized only if the B cells know their enemies and their structures very well. There are, however, millions of enemies (antigens) in nature.

This is like manufacturing a compatible key for each of millions of locks straight away. What is important is that the manufacturing agent does this without examining the lock or using any mould. It knows the formula by heart.

It is quite difficult for a human being to memorize the shape of even a single key. So, is it possible for a person to keep in mind the three-dimensional designs of millions of keys that are to open millions of locks?

Definitely not. However, a B cell so small as to be imperceptible by the eye keeps millions of bits of information in its memory, and uses them in correct combinations in a conscious way.

The storage of millions of formulae in a miniscule cell is a great miracle presented to man. No less miraculous is the cell's using this information to protect man's health.

It is obvious that the secret of the tremendous success of these tiny cells is beyond the boundaries of human's comprehension. Today, the power of the human mind even combined with advanced technology pales into insignificance in the face of the intelligence displayed by these cells. In fact, even evolutionist scientists cannot close their eyes to all these signs of intelligence, which are clear evidence of the existence of a conscious Creator. One of the greatest advocators of evolution in Turkey, Prof. Dr. Ali Demirsoy, confessed this in his book "*Inheritance and Evolution*":

> How and in what form did plasma cells obtain this information, and produce the antibody exclusively designed according to it? This question has not been answered precisely so far.[3]

As confessed by the evolutionist scientist above, how antibodies are produced is a point that has not been clearly understood as yet. The technology of the 20th century has proved insufficient even at the level of understanding the methods of this perfect production. In the years to come, as the methods used by these tiny cells — which are created to serve mankind — and how they implement them are unraveled, the perfection and artistry in the creation of these cells will be better understood.

The Structure of Antibodies

We have previously stated that antibodies are a type of protein. So, let us first examine the structure of proteins.

Proteins are made up of amino acids. Twenty different types of amino acids are arranged in different sequences to form different proteins. This is similar to making different necklaces by using beads in twenty different colours. The main differences among proteins are due to the sequence of these amino acids.

Yet there is an important point to remember: Any error in the amino acid sequence makes the protein useless, and even harmful. Therefore, there is no room for even the smallest error in the sequence.

So, how do the protein factories in the cell know in which sequence to arrange the amino acids they contain, and which protein to produce? The instructions for each of the thousands of different types of proteins are encoded in the genes found in the genetic data bank in the cell nucleus.

Therefore, these genes are required for the production of the antibodies which are a type of protein. There will be need for

There is a very important miracle here. There are only one hundred thousand genes in the human body compared to the 1.920.000 antibodies that are produced. This means that nine hundred thousand genes are missing.

Then how is it ever possible that such a small number of genes can produce antibodies about ten times their value? The miracle is revealed at this point. The cell combines the hundred thousand genes it contains in different combinations to form new antibodies. It receives the information from some genes and combines it with the information in other genes and makes the required production according to this combined information.

1,920,000 different antibodies are formed as a result of 5,200 different combinations.[4] This process represents a wisdom and planning that are too great for the human mind to comprehend, let alone design.

An unlimited number of combinations can be made with the use of one hundred thousand genes. The cell, however, uses, with great intelligence, only 5,200 basic combinations and produces 1,920,000 specific antibodies. How has the cell learned to make the right combinations out of these unlimited possibilities to form the required antibodies?

Making the correct combinations out of an infinite number of possibilities aside, how has the cell got this idea of making combinations?

Moreover, the produced combinations serve a certain purpose, and

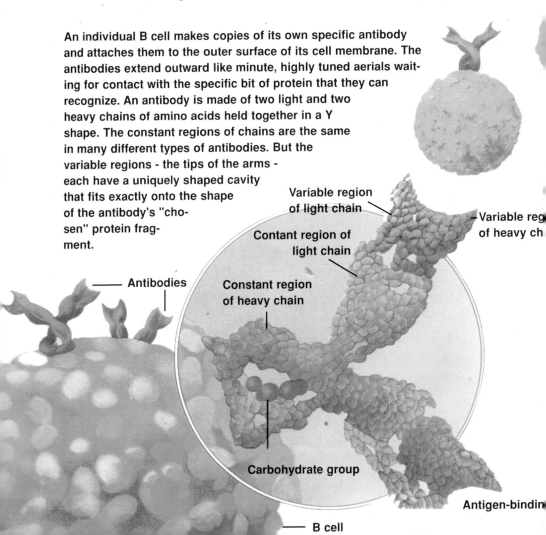

An individual B cell makes copies of its own specific antibody and attaches them to the outer surface of its cell membrane. The antibodies extend outward like minute, highly tuned aerials waiting for contact with the specific bit of protein that they can recognize. An antibody is made of two light and two heavy chains of amino acids held together in a Y shape. The constant regions of chains are the same in many different types of antibodies. But the variable regions - the tips of the arms - each have a uniquely shaped cavity that fits exactly onto the shape of the antibody's "chosen" protein fragment.

Antibodies

Variable region of light chain

Contant region of light chain

Variable reg of heavy ch

Constant region of heavy chain

Carbohydrate group

Antigen-bindin

B cell

aim to produce an antibody that would eliminate the antigen that enters the body. Therefore, the cell also knows the properties of the millions of antigens entering the body.

No intellect in this world can produce a design of such unparalleled perfection. But cells only the size of a hundredth of a millimeter can do so.

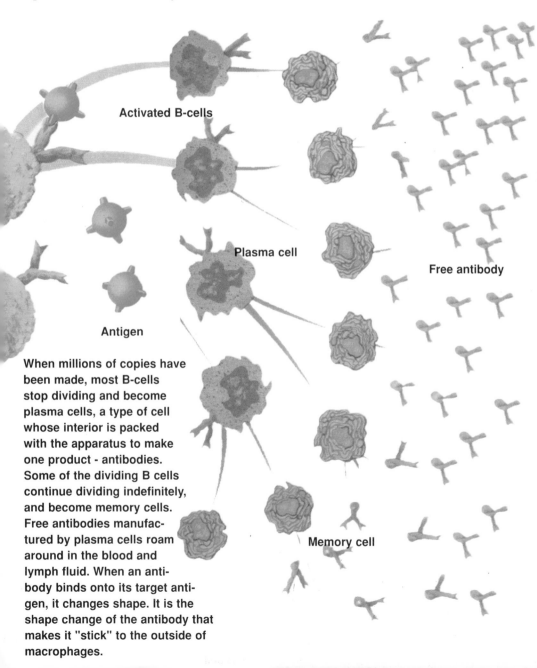

Activated B-cells

Plasma cell

Free antibody

Antigen

When millions of copies have been made, most B-cells stop dividing and become plasma cells, a type of cell whose interior is packed with the apparatus to make one product - antibodies. Some of the dividing B cells continue dividing indefinitely, and become memory cells. Free antibodies manufactured by plasma cells roam around in the blood and lymph fluid. When an antibody binds onto its target antigen, it changes shape. It is the shape change of the antibody that makes it "stick" to the outside of macrophages.

Memory cell

So, how has the cell learned such a special system?

The truth is that no cell has the opportunity to "learn" a biological function in the real sense. This is because the cell does not possess the ability to perform such an act at birth, nor has it the chance to develop the required skill during the rest of its lifetime. In such cases, it is a prerequisite that the system in the cell should be ready and complete at the beginning of life. The cell neither possesses the skill to learn such combinations, nor does it have the time to learn them, as this would cause it to fail in stopping the antigens entering the body and the body would lose the war.

The fact that a system that baffles mankind, even at the point of comprehending it, has been placed in a cell which has no ability to think and reason, has a very special meaning. This is the reflection of the uniqueness of the creation of Allah, the All-Knowing, in a tiny cell. In the Qur'an, it is stated that Allah's superior wisdom encompasses everything:

...They cannot grasp any of His knowledge save what He wills. His Footstool encompasses the heavens and the earth and their preservation does not tire Him. He is the Most High, the Magnificent. (Surat al-Baqara: 255)

If you were to design an antibody molecule, how would you do it? You would first have to carry out comprehensive research before deciding on the shape of the molecule. Surely you could not shape it randomly without an exact knowledge of its duty. Since the antibodies you are going to produce will make contact with antigens, you would have to be very well informed about the structure and specifications of the antigen, too.

Eventually, the antibody you will produce has to have a special and unique shape at one end. Only then can it bind to an antigen. The other end of it has to be similar to other antibodies. This is the only way the antigen destructing mechanism can be activated. As a result, one end has to be standard, while the other has to be different from the others (which come in more than one million different types).

Human beings, however, have been unable to design an antibody, despite all the technology at their disposal. The antibodies produced in the laboratory environment are either derived from antibody samples taken from the human body, or the bodies of other living beings.

Antibody Classes

We earlier stated that antibodies are a type of protein. These proteins, functioning in the defence of the body within the immune operation, are called "immune globulin" (a type of protein) and designated as "Ig".

The most characteristic proteins of the defence system, the immune globulin molecules bind to the antigens to inform other immune cells of the existence of the antigen or to start the destructive chain reactions of the war.

IgG (Immune Globulin G): IgG is the most common antibody. Its development takes only a few days, while its life span ranges from a few weeks to several years. IgGs circulate in the body and are mainly present in the blood, lymphatic system, and intestine. They circulate in the bloodstream, directly target the invader, and latch on to it as soon as they detect it. They have a strong antibacterial and antigen-destroying effect. They protect the body against bacteria and viruses, and neutralize the acidic property of toxins (poisons).

Additionally, the IgG may squeeze itself between cells, and eliminate the bacteria and micro-organic invaders that have infiltrated to the cells and the skin. Due their above-mentioned ability and small size, they can enter the placenta of a pregnant woman and protect an undefended foetus against possible infections.

If antibodies were not created with this characteristic which permits them to penetrate the placenta, the unborn child in the mother's womb would be unprotected against microbes. It would be under the threat of death even before it was born. For this reason, the antibodies of the mother protect the embryo against the enemies until the time of birth.

IgA (Immune Globulin A): These antibodies are present in sensitive regions where the body fights with antigens such as in tears, saliva, mother's milk, blood, air sacs, mucus, gastric and intestinal secretions. The sensitivity of those regions relates directly to the tendency of bacteria and viruses to prefer such damp mediums.

IgAs, which are structurally quite similar to each other, settle in those regions of the body where microbes are most likely to enter, and they keep this area under control. This is like placing reliable soldiers on guard at strategically critical points.

The antibodies, which protect the foetus from various diseases in the mother's womb, do not abandon the newborn following their birth, but continue to guard them. All newborn babies do need ongoing assistance from the mother, because there are no IgAs in the organism of a newborn baby. During this period, the IgAs present in the milk the baby sucks from its mother protect the baby's digestive system from the effect of many microbes. Just like IgGs, this antibody class also disappears after they have fulfilled their term of service, when the baby is a few weeks old.

Have you ever wondered who sends you these antibodies that try to protect you from microbes, when you are in the form of an embryo and unaware of anything? Is it your mother or your father? Or is it that they have taken a common decision and sent you these antibodies together? Certainly, the help in question is out of the control of both parents. The mother is not even aware that she has been endowed with such an aid plan. The father is just as unaware of all that is going on.

Then why do the cells present in the mother's breast and productive of these antibodies function in such a way? Which power has told these cells that the newborn needs antibodies? It is by no means a coincidence that the cells engaging in antibody production for the baby are located in the place where the newborns suckle.

Here, there is another very important miracle. Antibodies are protein-structured organisms. Proteins, on the other hand, are digested in the human stomach. Therefore, normally, the baby suckling milk from its mother would digest these antibodies in its stomach, and would become unprotected against microbes. The stomach of the newborn baby, however, is created in such a way that it does not digest and destroy these antibodies. The production of protein-digesting enzymes is very little at this stage. Therefore, antibodies vital for life are not digested and they protect the newborn baby from its enemies.

The miracle does not end here. The antibodies, which are not broken down by the stomach, can, however, be absorbed by the intestine as a whole. The intestinal cells of the newborn are created in such a way as to do so.

Unquestionably, it is no coincidence that these miraculous events are arranged in such a sequence. The human body, a meticulously planned example of creation, passes from the embryonic stage to having a fully functional immune system in a perfectly phased manner. This is because the events that are supposed to take place in the body every day, every hour and every minute, are computed in an extremely finely-tuned manner. Certainly, the author of this precise calculation is Allah, Who creates everything according to a very intricate plan.

IgM (Immune globulin M): These antibodies are present in the blood, lymph and on the surface of the B cells. When the human organism encounters an antigen, IgM is the first antibody that is produced in the body in response to this enemy.

An unborn child can produce IgMs in the sixth month of gestation. If an enemy ever attacks the baby in the mother's womb, for example, if it infects it with a microbial disease, the baby's IgM production will increase. In order to determine whether the foetus has been infected with a disease or not, the IgM level in its blood is measured.

IgD (Immune globulin D): IgDs are also present in the blood, lymph, and on the surface of B cells. They are not capable of acting independently. By attaching themselves to the surfaces of T cells, they help them capture antigens.

IgE (Immune globulin E): IgEs are antibodies circulating in the bloodstream. These antibodies, which are responsible for calling fighter and some other blood cells to war, also cause some allergic reactions in the body. For this reason, the level of IgE is high in allergic bodies.

Evolutionists' Attempts to Cover Up The Evidence of Creation

First, let us review the information we have examined so far:

- Antibodies latch on to antigens (enemies) entering the body.

- A different type of antibody is produced for every enemy.

- The cell is able to produce thousands of different antibodies for thousands of different antigens.

- This production starts as soon as the enemy enters the body and is identified.

- There is full harmony between the antigen and the three dimensional antibody, which is produced for that specific antigen, just as a key exactly fits a lock.

- The cell, when required, arranges the information it possesses in a conscious way and produces different antibodies.

- While doing all this, it displays wisdom and planning far beyond the boundaries of the human mind's comprehension.

- Certain antibodies, which are specially placed in the mother's milk, meet the antibody need of a baby, which is as yet unable to produce these antibodies.

- The baby's stomach does not digest the antibodies, but spares them so that they serve the baby's body.

Here we see a perfectly working system in place. Inside the cells that produce the antibodies, Allah placed information containing the construction plans of these antibodies that would fill thousands of encyclopaedia pages. Furthermore, He has given these unconscious cells the ability to make combinations, such as are beyond the reach of the human mind.

How do people who blindly believe in evolution explain the existence of such a perfect system? The answer is very simple: they cannot.

The only thing they do is put forward illogical assumptions which strongly self-contradict. There are many imaginary scenarios without any scientific validity that are solely directed towards finding an answer to the question of "How can we explain this system in terms of evolution?".

The most popular of these scenarios maintains that the immune system evolved from a single antibody. Here is the summary of this scenario which has no scientific basis:

*Initially the defence system comprised of a single gene that produced a single type of immunoglobulin (a kind of protein). But this gene **"rapidly created copies of itself (!)"** and **developed** these copies so that they formed a different molecule of immunoglobulin. Then the control mechanisms **developed** that monitor the manufacturing of different genes which possess the ability to re-combine".*

This example is important in seeing how shaky are the grounds the theory of evolution is built on, and in understanding the brainwashing and window-dressing methods evolutionists frequently have recourse to. Now let us examine this deceit sentence by sentence:

Sentence 1: "Initially the defence system comprised of a single gene that produced a single type of immunoglobulin (a kind of protein)."

The first question that must be asked is:

"By whom was this inaugural gene created?"

Evolutionists try to present this stage as an insignificant detail and circumvent it. However, how this initial gene has originated must be explained. It is scientifically impossible for a gene to have formed by itself. The impossibility of the coincidental formation of the gene sequence is a fact which has been admitted by evolutionist scientists many times. We can give an example from Prof. Ali Demirsoy, a Turkish evolutionist, on this subject.

*That is, if life requires a certain sequence, it can be said that this has a probability likely to be realised once in the whole universe. Otherwise some **metaphysical powers** beyond our definition must have acted in its formation.*[5]

Yet evolutionists cover up this point and make a senseless presupposition such as "whatever the argument, there surely was a gene at the beginning." As is quite evident, the scenario collapses right at the first step.

Sentence 2: "But this gene "rapidly created copies of itself (!)" and developed these copies so that they formed a different molecule of immunoglobulin."

Though impossible, let us suppose that there was a gene at the beginning. Though it is utterly impossible for this first gene to have formed by itself, evolutionists make statements, lacking any logical basis such as "it created copies of itself." Such statements, which have no scientific value, constitute a good example of the window-dressing style of the evolutionists. A hypothesis assuming that a gene created and developed different copies of itself complies neither with the rules of logic nor with scientific facts.

Moreover, the antibodies produced by such an imaginary gene, which has supposedly formed by itself, and its copies, have to possess such properties and structure as will stop the antigens coming from the external world. This means that the same Creator, that is, Allah created both antigens and the genes that are responsible for producing antibodies for antigens.

Sentence 3: "Then the control mechanisms developed that manage the manufacturing of different genes which possess the ability to re-combine."

Unable to explain even the working principles of these control and combination mechanisms, evolutionists evade the issue by saying that "this system brought itself into being" whenever it serves their purpose. They do not attempt to describe how such an incredible system developed by itself as a result of coincidences. When they try to bring some explanations of their own to these issues, they cannot put forward anything but fabricated and ridiculous scenarios. By doing so, they expose their weakness, and the unreasonableness of the claim they make.

So great is the wisdom displayed in these control mechanisms that approximately two million differently structured products are fabricated from thousands of combinations of units of information. Yet, as mentioned before, neither the cell, nor any system within the cell has the ability to "learn" and "develop". Moreover, the cell makes these information combinations by selecting only the right ones out of infinite possibilities. Therefore, this requires a much more conscious and reasonable selecting. mechanism.

Those who make such a claim may well advance the following theories for any given product that is manufactured by technology or the human mind:

"Stone tablets created themselves and later developed into computers on their own.". Or,

"Kites that have created themselves later developed into jet planes."

The above sentences would sound absolutely absurd to any national person. However, even these sentences are much more logical than saying that the elements of the defence system, the working principles of which have not even been discovered, emerged by coincidence.

What is more, the presence of antibodies alone is not sufficient to protect the human body. For the defence system to operate, and for the human being to survive, macrophages, helper T cells, killer T cells, suppressor T cells, memory cells, B cells and many other factors must work in cooperation.

ORGANS EMPLOYED IN DEFENCE

Warrior Production Centre: The Bone Marrow

When atom bombs were dropped on Hiroshima and Nagasaki, many people exposed to the radiation released by the explosions died 10 or 15 days later from internal bleeding or infection. Animal experiments conducted to explore what happened to such casualties revealed that whole-body radiation kills the generative cells in blood-forming and lymphoid organs. Without the cells responsible for clotting and for fighting invaders, the body dies.[6]

The factory of these vital cells is the bone marrow. The interesting point is that many diverse products are produced in this factory. Some of

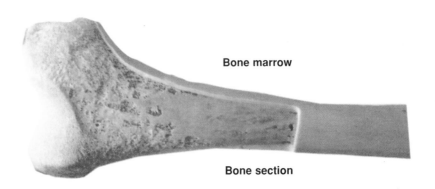

Bone marrow

Bone section

the cells produced here play a role in the production of phagocytes, some in the coagulation
of blood, some in the decomposition of substances. These cells differ in function just as they differ in their structure.

It is remarkable that a very special production system has been established for many different cells that work towards the same goal.

Here, there seems to be an impregnable
barrier for the theory of evolution. This is be-

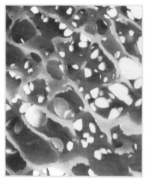

Bone marrow

cause the theory of evolution claims that multi-celled organisms have
evolved from one-celled organisms.

So, how can coincidentally formed cells build a system capable of
producing new cells in the very structure they have constituted? This is
similar to thousands of bricks, which have burst into the air as a result of
an explosion at a brick factory, having fallen down on top of each other by
chance and, in the process, making a brand new building. Moreover, in
this building there must also be another factory to build new bricks.

It has to be remembered that the creation of a human body is a million times superior to that of a building. The cell, which is the building
block of the body, has a design too perfect to be compared with any man-
made product. This analogy between the cell and the brick has simply
been made in order to clarify how deceitful the hypothesis of evolutionists is.

The Faculty in Us: The Thymus

On biological examination, the thymus would seem to be an ordinary organ without any particular function. The work it does, however,
when studied in detail, is quite unbelievable.

In the thymus, the lymphocytes get some sort of training. No, you
have not misread this. The cells receive training in the thymus.

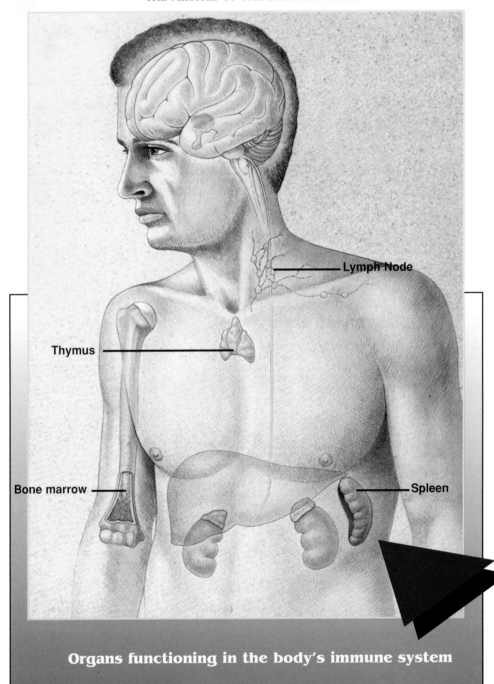

Lymph Node

Thymus

Bone marrow

Spleen

Organs functioning in the body's immune system

Training is an information transfer, which can be exercised on beings with a certain level of intelligence. So there is an important point that needs mention here. What gives the training is a lump of meat, which is the thymus, and what receives it is a miniscule cell. In the last analysis, both are unconscious beings.

At the end of this training, lymphocytes are equipped with a very important body of information. They learn to identify the particular characteristics of the cells in the body. In some sense, the lymphocytes are taught the identities of the body cells. Finally, these cells leave the thymus loaded with information.

Thus, as the lymphocytes function in the body, they do not attack the cells, the identity of which they have been taught. Any other cell or foreign matter is attacked and destroyed by them.

For years, the thymus was considered to be a vestigial organ by evolutionist scientists and used as so-called evidence for evolution. In recent years, however, it has been revealed that this organ constitutes the wellspring of our defence system. After this was understood, evolutionists,

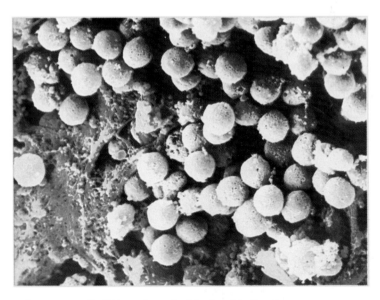

Immune cells (T lymphocytes) trained in the thymus.

who once proclaimed the thymus to be a vestigial organ, now advanced a totally opposite theory for the same organ. They claimed that the thymus did not exist before, and originated through gradual evolution. They still maintain that the thymus formed in a longer evolutionary period than many organs. However, without the thymus, or without its being fully developed, T cells could not have learned to identify the enemy and the defence system would not have functioned. Someone without such a system would not survive. Even your reading this sentence now is proof that the thymus was not created through a long evolutionary process, but has always existed, perfect and intact in all respects, since the advent of the first human being.

A Versatile Organ: The Spleen

Another wondrous element of our defence system is the spleen. The spleen is made up of two parts: red pulp and white pulp. The fresh lymphocytes produced in the white pulp are first transferred to the red pulp and then join in the blood stream. A detailed study of the operations carried out in this organ, which is dark red in colour and located high up the abdomen reveals an extraordinary picture. Its quite difficult and complicated functions are what make it so wonderful and extraordinary.

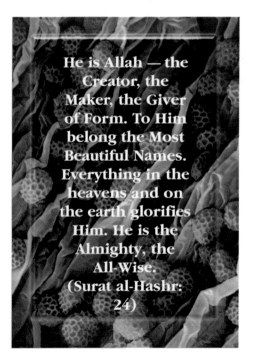

He is Allah — the Creator, the Maker, the Giver of Form. To Him belong the Most Beautiful Names. Everything in the heavens and on the earth glorifies Him. He is the Almighty, the All-Wise. (Surat al-Hashr: 24)

The duties of the spleen, such as contributing to cell production, phagocytosis, conservation of red blood cells, and immunity construction, are at least as important as they are difficult. Certainly, the spleen is a lump of meat just like all our other organs. Yet it displays a performance and a degree of intelligence unexpected from a lump of meat. It organizes everything, not allowing any problems to occur, and works without rest. Indeed, the spleen works strenuously for the human from the moment of his birth, and continues its function as long as Allah wills.

Cell Production

The bone marrow of the baby in the mother's womb is not entirely able to fulfill its function of producing blood cells. The bone marrow can perform this function only after birth. Would the baby be anaemic in the meantime?

No. At this stage, the spleen comes into play and takes control. Sensing that the body needs red blood cells, thrombocytes, and granulocytes, the spleen starts to produce these cells in addition to lymphocytes, which is its main duty.

The spleen, however, is an unconscious lump of meat. It is not capable of assuming such a responsibility. Besides, even if it did, how would it be equipped with the required information and components to produce the extremely complex cells and proteins? Allah, Who created the human body, created the spleen in such a way as to enable it to take on other responsibilities in addition its own task when necessary, and equipped it with the necessary stimulus and production systems.

Phagocytosis

The spleen contains a large number of macrophages (cleaner cells). These engulf and digest old and damaged red blood cells, some damaged blood cells and some substances that are carried to the spleen through the blood.

There is a very important chemical recycling system at work here.

The macrophage cells in the spleen convert the haemoglobin protein, which is found in the composition of the red blood cells they have engulfed, to bilirubin, a bile pigment. Then, the bilirubin is released to the venous circulation and sent to the liver. In this form, it can be discharged out of the body along with the bile. However, the iron molecule found in the bilirubin which is about to be discharged out of the intestines along with the bile, is a rare material which is very valuable for the body. For this reason, iron is absorbed back in a certain region of the small intestines and from there, it first goes to the liver and then to the bone marrow. Here, the purpose is both to discharge the bilirubin, which is a harmful substance, and, at the same time, to regain the iron.

The bilirubin balance is crucial for our body. This is because even the slightest problem in this system would lead to serious outcomes. One of the best examples is that when bilirubin goes above a certain level, jaundice develops in the body. However, the cells in our body, as if they are aware of this danger, discharge the harmful materials from our body with a great precision while they select the useful ones among them and put them into use once again.

Red Blood Cell Storage

The skills of the spleen do not end here. The spleen stores a certain amount of blood cells (red blood cell and thrombocytes). The word "store" may conjure up an image of a separate compartment in the spleen that can be used for storage. The spleen, however, is a small organ, and it has no space to use as a storage room. In such cases, the spleen expands to make room for red blood cells and thrombocytes. A spleen enlarged due to some diseases may also have an enlarged storage space.

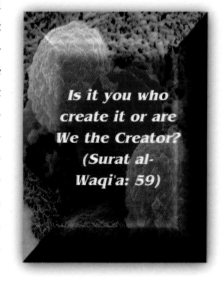

Is it you who create it or are We the Creator? (Surat al-Waqi'a: 59)

Contribution To War

When a microbial infection or any other malady develops in the body, the body mounts a defensive attack on this enemy, prodding the warrior cells to multiply. At such moments, the spleen enhances lymphocyte and macrophage production. Thus, the spleen also participates in the "emergency operation" that is launched at times when disease could harm the human body.

Another Production Centre: The Lymph Nodes

In the human body, there is a police force and a police intelligence organization scattered throughout the body. In this system, there are also police stations which have policemen on guard, and which produce new policemen when required.

This system is the lymphatic system and the police stations are the lymph nodes. The policemen of the system are lymphocytes.

The lymphatic system as it stands is a miracle performed for the benefit of mankind. This system comprises of lymphatic vessels that are diffused throughout the body, lymph nodes that are located at certain spots on these vessels, the lymphocytes produced by lymph nodes, which patrol in the lymphatic vessels, and the lymph fluid circulating in the lymphatic vessels in which lymphocytes swim.

The system works as follows: The lymph fluid in the lymphatic vessels spread throughout the body makes contact with the tissues located around the capillary lymphatic vessels. The lymph fluid that returns to the lymphatic vessels right after this contact brings along some information about these tissues. These pieces of information are transmitted to the nearest lymph node located on the lymphatic vessels. If any hostile action has started in the tissues, its knowledge is forwarded to the lymph node through the lymph fluid.

In case any danger is sensed following the examination of the nature of the enemy, an alarm is given. At this point, the rapid production of lymphocytes and some other warrior cells starts in the lymph nodes.

After the production stage, the new soldiers are transported to the front where the battle is fought. These new soldiers will travel from the lymph nodes to the lymphatic vessels through the lymph fluid. The soldiers, which are diffused into the blood stream from the lymphatic vessels, finally reach the battleground. This is why the lymph nodes in the infected region swell first. This shows that the lymphocyte production has increased in that region.

Now, let us summarize the system:

- A special transportation system that covers the length and breadth of body.

- Lymph node stations dispersed throughout different regions of the body.

- The intelligence operation directed at the enemy cells.

- Production of soldiers according to the results of the intelligence report.

It is impossible for this system, which would collapse in the absence of even one of its elements, to have originated by developing gradually over time. For instance, a system with lymph nodes and lymphocytes, but without lymphatic vessels, would not be of any use. The system can work properly only if all its elements are created simultaneously.

CELLS ON DUTY IN THE SYSTEM

I f an enemy overcomes all barriers and succeeds in entering our body, this does not mean that the defence army has been defeated. On the contrary, the real war has just begun, and the main soldiers come into play at this stage. The first soldiers to meet the foe are the eater cells, that is, phagocytes, which continuously travel in our body and keep control of what is going on.

These are "special cleaning cells", which ingest the unwanted microbes that have penetrated the inner surfaces of the body, and alert the defence system when necessary.

Certain cells in the defence system capture, break down, digest, and eliminate the miniscule particles and liquid foreign matter that have entered our body. This event is called "phagocytosis". (cell engulfing)

Phagocytosis is one of the most important elements of the immune system. It provides an immediate and effective protection against infections.

Phagocytes, considered the "police forces of the body," can be examined under two separate headings.

1. Mobile police forces: These roam in the blood and shuttle forwards and backwards between the tissues when required. These cell units, which circulate throughout the body, also serve as scavengers.

2. Immobile police forces: These are immobile macrophages, which

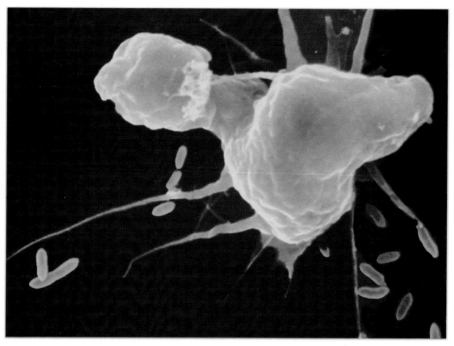

Phagocytosis in progress. The macrophage (yellow) while digesting the bacteria (blue).

are situated in the gaps in various tissues. They perform phagocytosis on the micro-organisms from where they are, without moving.

If the invader antigens (foreign micro-organisms) are few enough for the present eater cells to deal with, they are destroyed with no extra alarm being given. But if the invader microbes are too great in number, the eater cells may fail to get them under control. Unable to digest all of them, they expand in size. When distended by the antigens, the cells burst, causing a liquid substance (pus) to overflow. This does not mean that the war is lost. So far, the eater cells have just met the microbes, which have still many tougher barriers to pass. The formation of pus activates the lymphocytes, which have been delivered from the bone marrow, the lymph nodes, and above all, the thymus. In a second wave of defence, the newly arriving defence cells attack everything they find around, including cell debris, available antigens, and even old white blood cells. These defence cells are the real eater cells, — the macrophages, a type of phagocyte.

The First Aid Forces: The Macrophages

When the war becomes intense, the macrophages swing into action. Macrophages operate in a specific manner exclusive to themselves. They do not become involved in a one-to-one combat like the antibodies. Unlike the antibodies, they do not work with a system similar to a bomb aimed at a single target. Just like a gun firing lead shot, or a bomb that can be aimed at many targets together, the macrophages can destroy a great number of enemies together, all at the same time.

Like all other defence cells, the macrophages are also derived from the bone marrow. The macrophages, which have a very long life span, can live for months, and even years. Despite their small size (10-15 micrometers), they are highly crucial for human life. They possess the ability to absorb and digest big molecules in the cell through phagocytosis (ingestion).

Their characteristic of ingestion makes them the scavengers of the defence system. They remove all materials that need to be cleaned up, such as micro-organisms, antigen-antibody complexes, and other substances similar in structure to an antigen. At the end of these processes, substances that would be qualified as antigens are digested, and thus pose no further threat to the organism.

General Alarm

When a country is involved in war, a general mobilization is declared. Most of the natural resources and the budget are expended on military requirements. The economy is re-arranged to meet the needs of this extraordinary situation and the country is involved in an all-out war effort. Similarly, the defence system would also announce mass mobilization, recruiting all of its elements to fight the enemy. Do you wonder how this happens?

If enemy members are more than the currently fighting macrophages can handle, a special substance is secreted. The name of this substance is "pyrogen" and it is a kind of alarm call.

After traveling a long way, "pyrogen" reaches the brain where it stimulates the fever-increasing centre of the brain. Once alerted, the brain sets off alarms in the body and the person develops a high fever. The patient with a high fever naturally feels the need to rest. Thus, the energy needed by the defence army is not spent elsewhere. The pyrogen produced by the macrophages is perfectly designed to trigger the fever-raising mechanism of the brain. Therefore, the macrophage, and the pyrogen, and the temperature-raising centre of the brain, and the brain have all to be created at the same time.

As is evident, there is a perfect plan at work. Every requirement is created flawlessly for this plan to succeed; the macrophages, the pyrogen substance and other similar substances, the fever-raising centre of the brain and the fever-raising mechanisms of the body...

In the absence of even one of these, the system would simply not work. Therefore, it can by no means be claimed that such a system could have originated step by step through evolution.

Who, then, has made this plan?

Who knows that the body's fever must rise, and that only that way the energy needed by the defence army will not be spent elsewhere?

Is it the macrophages?

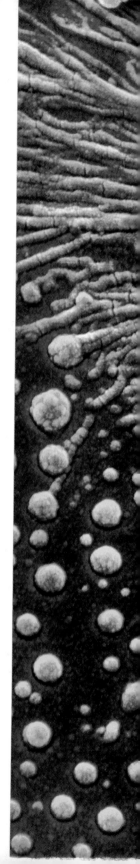

To the right, you can see macrophages while trying to ingest foreign materials.

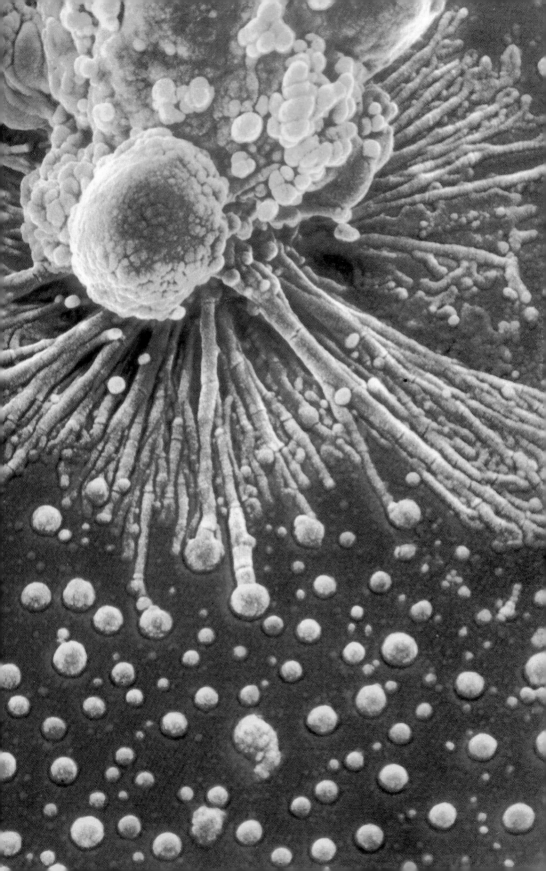

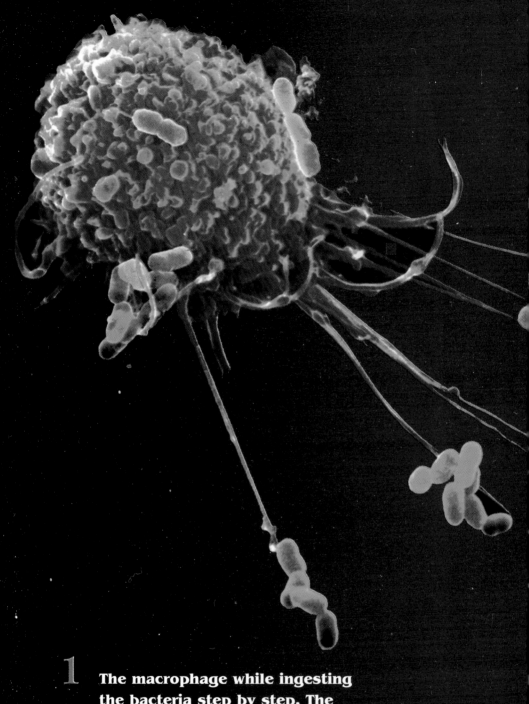

1 The macrophage while ingesting the bacteria step by step. The macrophage extends forward to capture the bacteria.

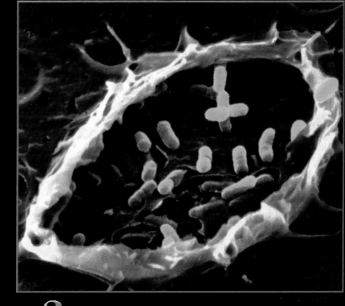

2 The bacteria are captured and trapped within the extensions of the macrophage membrane.

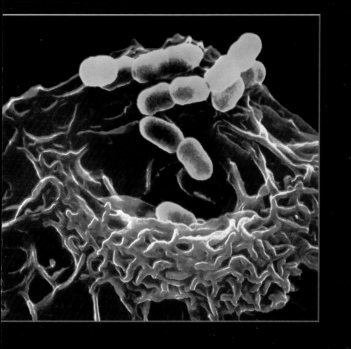

3 The bacteria, which are trapped in the macrophage membrane, are absorbed one by one.

Macrophages are merely tiny cells invisible to the naked eye. They do not have the capacity to think. They are living organisms that only obey an established superior order; they merely carry out their duties.

Is it the brain?

Definitely no. Nor does the brain possess any power to create or produce something. Just as in all other systems, in this system, too, it is in a position not to give orders, but to obey orders and submit to them.

Is it man?

Certainly not. This system protects man from certain death, although he is not even aware that such a perfect system is at work in his own body. Even if man were ever ordered to develop an army in his own body to fight the enemy and cause his fever to rise, and provide this army to work round the clock in his entire body, he would simply have no idea what to do.

Today, mankind is not even able to understand the details of the present order in the defence system, despite all the technology at its disposal — much less imitate it.

It is an obvious fac that man was created with all of his features in place. Willingly or unwillingly, he submits to his Creator and the systems He established. Just as everything else does…

…No, everything in the heavens and earth belongs to Him. Everything is obedient to Him. (Surat al-Baqara: 116)

Information Transfer

Another incredible function of the macrophages is supplying the lymphocytes, i.e., the B and T cells, which are the real heroes of the defence system, with information about the enemy. After phagocytosing the antigen, the antigen-presenting cells go to the lymph nodes (lymphatic tissue) through the lymphatic channels.

This is a very important detail. Only if a cell possesses consciousness and reason can it be capable of supplying and forwarding the information

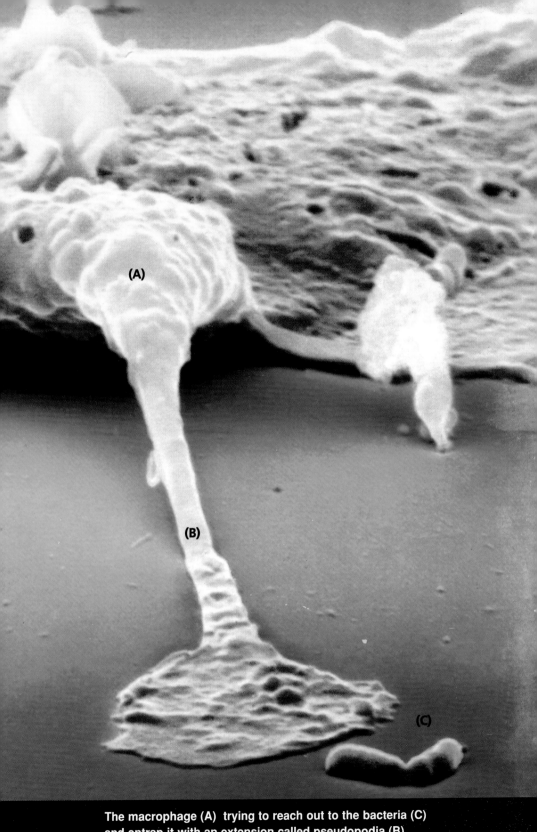

The macrophage (A) trying to reach out to the bacteria (C) and entrap it with an extension called pseudopodia (B).

pertaining to an enemy to the relevant centres. For the macrophage cell to know that this information will be processed by the lymphocytes, it has to be perfectly informed about the general strategy of the defence system. It is very clear that the macrophage, just like all the other cells, is the obedient element of a totally integrated system.

Top Heroes: The Lymphocytes

The lymphocytes are the main cells of the defence system. The intense war in the body can only be won with the strenuous efforts of the lymphocytes. The life stories of these cells are full of incredibly interesting and wonderful stages, each of which, standing alone, is enough to demonstrate the decrepit nature of the theory of evolution.

These bold warriors are present in the bone marrow, lymph nodes, salivary glands, spleen, tonsils and joints. The lymphocytes are primarily present and produced in the bone marrow.

The formation of lymphocyte in the bone marrow is one of the most mysterious events of biology. Here, stem cells rapidly pass through a number of biological stages and take on a completely new structure by turning into lymphocytes. (A stem cell is an unspecialized cell that gives rise to a specific specialized cell, such as a blood cell.) When it is considered that, despite the great developments in genetic engineering, the transformation of even the plainest microbe species into other similar species is considered impossible, the mystery of this event, which takes place in the bone marrow, becomes even greater. This mystery, unsolved by science to date, is a very simple process for our body. For this reason, many evolutionist scientists have confessed that natural selection or mutation tales cannot account for the mystery in such a transformation. Prof. Dr. Ali Demirsoy stated that a complex cell like the lymphocyte, which carries almost all the responsibility of the war, could not have evolved from a simple cell:

Complex cells have never been generated from primitive cells through an ev-

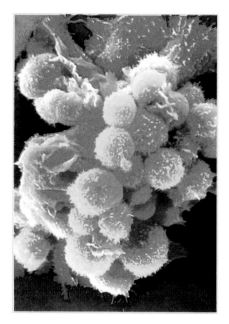

Lymphocytes at war (yellow), fighting with cancer cells.

olutionary process as recently suggested. [7]

This fact is actually very well known by the scientists of our day. Yet, obviously, when they accept this fact, they will equally be obliged to accept the existence of a Creator. This is something which most of them are very reluctant to do.

The world renowned biochemist Michael J. Behe states that evolutionists disregard some facts for the sake of denying the being of Allah:

Also, and unfortunately, too often criticisms have been dismissed by the scientific community for fear of giving ammunition to creationists. It is ironic that in the name of protecting science, trenchant scientific criticism of natural selection has been brushed aside. [8]

Lymphocytes, the products of this mysterious transformation, which is one of the facts ignored, play a very interesting role in the defence system. They check on the body cells several times a day to see if there are any sick cells. If they find any sick or old cells, they destroy them. There are almost 100 trillion cells in our body and lymphocytes make up only 1%.

Now, imagine a country having an exceedingly high population, around 100 trillion. The number of health care workers (lymphocytes) would then be 1 trillion. If we think that the world's current population is some 7 billion, the number of the people living in our imaginary country would be almost 14 million 285 thousand times the world's population. Would it be possible for all the members of a country with such a high population to have a check-up one by one, and moreover, several times in the same day?

You will surely say no, but this process is carried out in your body every day; lymphocytes roam throughout your body several times a day to do a health check.

Is it possible to attribute the extremely organized operation of such a great mass of living beings to coincidence?

Can coincidences account for each one of a trillion lymphocytes assuming such an arduous and demanding task?

Certainly not!

Allah, the Lord of all Worlds, created each one of these one trillion lymphocytes and charged them with the responsibility of protecting man.

Lymphocytes play a very important role against major infectious diseases such as AIDS, cancer, rabies and tuberculosis, and serious ailments such as angina and rheumatism. Of course, this does not mean that lymphocytes do not have any role to play with other diseases. Even the common cold is nothing but a combat fought by the lymphocytes to keep those very dangerous common cold viruses away from the body.

The human body can defeat many of its enemies by using antibodies. This may lead you to wonder why lymphocytes intervene in the war directly when they already make a considerable contribution by producing antibodies. However, some microbes are so deadly that very strong chemical toxins are needed for their removal. Therefore, some lymphocytes use these chemical toxins and directly participate in the war.

How then would the defence system stop these enemies?

First, chemists and a laboratory would be needed to produce the toxin. The structure of the required material is too special to be formed by coincidence. Allah, Who knows that the human body will face such an enemy, or rather, Who created such an enemy for man to take warning, has also given the lymphocytes to synthesize this toxin.

So, is this chemical material satisfactory?

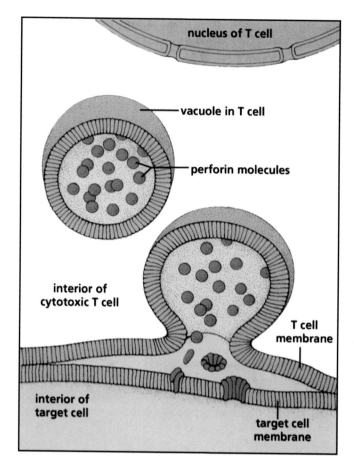

nucleus of T cell

vacuole in T cell

perforin molecules

interior of
cytotoxic T cell

T cell
membrane

interior of
target cell

target cell
membrane

In immune individuals, killer T cells attack and destroy cells bearing a foreign antigen, such as virus-infected or cancerous cells. These T cells have storage vacuoles that contain a chemical called perforin because it perforates cell membranes. During the killing process, the vacuoles in a T cell fuse with the cell membrane and release units of the protein perforin. These units combine to form pores in the target membrane. Thereafter, fluid and salts enter so that the target cell eventually bursts.

No, because this substance cannot freely circulate in the blood, as this would mean the death of our own cells as well.

How then will this toxin be used without causing any harm to our cells?

The answer to this question is hidden in the perfection of the creation of the lymphocytes. Toxins are placed in sacs located in the cell membrane of the lymphocytes. This helps the chemical weapon to be used easily. The lymphocyte injects this toxin only when it contacts the enemy cell, eventually killing it.

The lymphocytes come in two types: B cells and T cells.

The Weapon Factories of the Human Body:

The B Cells

Some of the lymphocytes produced in the bone marrow depart when they mature and become fully functional, and are transported to the lymphatic tissues through the blood. These lymphocytes are called the B cells.

B cells are the weapon factories of the body and they produce the proteins, called antibodies, which are meant to attack the enemy.

The B Cell Pathway

The cells undergo a highly complex and laborious process to become B cells. These cells must first pass a severe test in order to become the warriors who will protect human health.

In their initial phase, the B cells rearrange the gene fragments that will form an antibody molecule. These genes are actively transcribed as soon as the rearrangement is complete. At this point, it is very important to note how a tiny cell can perform complex tasks such as arranging and transcription. What is arranged and transcribed is actually information. And information can be arranged and organized only by a being who possesses intelligence. Furthermore, the outcome after the arrangement is

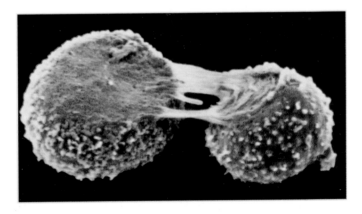

A B cell during division

extremely important: this information will later be used in the manufacture of antibodies.

The transformation of B cells rapidly goes on. Upon an order coming
from an unknown source, cells produce proteins called "alfa" and "beta",
which surround the cell membrane. At a further level, a range of complicated processes are due to take place in the cell to enable it to produce
some molecules that will enable it to bind to antigens. At the end of all
these complicated operations, the cells turn into a factory that recognizes
the enemy as soon as it makes contact with it, and is able produce millions
of different weapons.

Can Every B Cell That Has Been Manufactured Stay Alive?

The more we delve into the details of the defence system, the more
miracles we encounter. As stated before, B cells manufacture antibodies.
Antibodies are weapons that are manufactured purely to cause harm to
enemy cells. So, what happens if the weapons produced by the B cell con-
fuse their targets and start to hit friendly cells?

In that case, the other cells send a signal inside the B cell. This signal
is actually an order for the cell to "commit suicide". Eventually, some enzymes in the nucleus of the cell are activated and they decompose the
DNA of the cell. A perfectly working auto-control mechanism protects the
body, and finally, only the B cells that produce antibodies that cause harm
to the enemy can stay alive.

Only comprised of a compact nucleus and very little cytoplasm initially, the B cells undergo unbelievable changes when they meet an antigen. They divide repeatedly and build up thousands of assembly points in
their cytoplasm for the manufacture of antibodies, as well as an extensive
channeling system for the packaging and exporting the antibodies. One B
cell can pump out more than 10 million antibody molecules an hour.

Here is a single cell that transforms itself into a factory competent enough to produce 10 million weapons an hour on meeting an enemy. If we remember that this cell can produce different weapons for each of its millions of enemies, we can better understand the scope of the miracle in question here.

Some B cells become "memory cells". These cells do not immediately participate in the body's defence, but keep molecular records of past invaders in order to accelerate a potential war in the future. Their memory is very strong. When the body meets the same enemy again, this time it is rapidly geared to the appropriate weaponry production. Thus, defence becomes faster and more efficient.

Here, we cannot help asking ourselves: "How can man, who considers himself the most advanced being, have a memory weaker than that of a tiny cell?"

Unable to explain even how the memory of a normal human being forms and works, evolutionists never attempt to explain the existence of such a memory as a matter of evolution.

If a lump of flesh the size of a hundredth of a millimeter had only one single piece of information, and used this information for the benefit of mankind in the most accurate way, even this would be a miracle in its own right. However, what we are referring to here goes far beyond that. The cell stores millions of pieces of information for the benefit of man and uses this information accurately in combinations beyond man's comprehension. Man is able to survive thanks to the wisdom these cells display.

Memory cells are cells specially created to protect man's health. Allah equipped them with strong memorizing ability by design. Otherwise, it would be impossible for the cell to develop a strategy on its own accord and give itself within this strategy the responsibility for storing information. Moreover, the cell is even unaware of such a need; much less does it feel the need to employ such a strategy.

In addition, there is another important question that needs to be answered about the strong memories of the memory cells. In a normal human being, eight million cells die every second to be replaced by new ones. Therefore, the metabolism continuously renews itself. Yet the life span of memory cells is much longer than the life span of other cells. This characteristic helps them to protect people from diseases thanks to the information in their memories. These cells, however, are not everlasting. Though a long time later, they eventually die. At this point, we are left with a very surprising situation. Memory cells transfer the information they possess to the next generation before they die. People are indebted to these memory cells for not having to be afflicted all over again by the same in diseases they caught in infancy (measles, mumps, etc.).

How then can this cell know that it has to transfer this information?

This surely cannot be attributed to the cell itself, but to the ability granted to it by its Creator.

How Do the B cells Recognize the Enemy?

In a complete state of preparedness for war, the B cells then learn to discriminate the enemies from the body cells before defending the body.

They do not need to expend much effort to do this, because these cells and the antibodies they manufacture are able to recognize the enemy directly from their shapes without any assistance. A receptor on their surface meets the antigen for which it was programmed, and binds to several small parts on it. Thus, the antigen is identified as a foreigner. In this way, B cells can easily recognize antigens, such as bacteria.

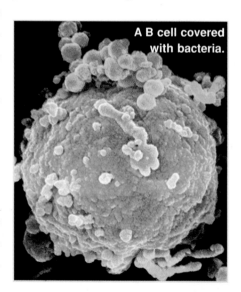

A B cell covered with bacteria.

What is the Function of B cells?

B cells are like guards who are always on the look-out for microbes. When they encounter an in-

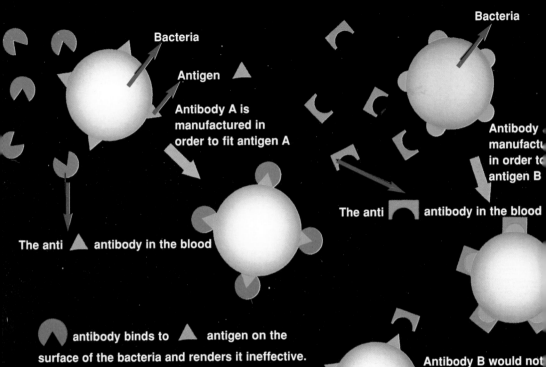

Bacteria

Antigen

Antibody A is manufactured in order to fit antigen A

Bacteria

Antibody manufactu in order to antigen B

The anti ▲ antibody in the blood

The anti antibody in the blood

antibody binds to ▲ antigen on the surface of the bacteria and renders it ineffective.

Antibody B would not fit antigen A

Antibodies with different antigens cannot be effective against bacteri

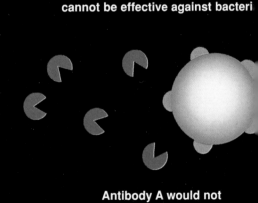

Antibody A would not fit antigen B

Bacteria and viruses carry chemicals on their surfaces called antigens. Some lymphocytes produce antibodies to bind themselves to antigens, thus enabling the white cell to easily ingest the bacteria. Antibodies have distinct features and they only bind to antigens for which they are produced. As illustrated in the above picture, a triangular antigen perfectly fits to an antibody, which has a triangular cut. (top left). Yet the same antibody (bottom) does not fit to a round antigen.

vader, they rapidly divide and start to produce antibodies. These antibodies bind to microbes like B cell receptors. The enemy cells that are marked by the antibodies as foreigners are driven out of the body at the end of the relentless struggle of phagocytes and T cells. By the time the B cells inactivate the enemy with the millions of antibodies they have produced, they have also marked it for killer cells. Here, there is another important point, which is as important as destroying and marking foreign cells. It is about how so many antibodies can be produced by a limited number of genes.

As outlined in detail in the section on "Antibodies", the B cells use the genes in the human body to manufacture antibodies. However, the number of genes in the human body is less than the number of antibodies produced. This situation causes no problem for the cells. Despite all these limitations, they succeed in producing nearly 2 million antibody types an hour.[9] B cells interact in various combinations with available genes to make the above-mentioned production. It is literally impossible for a cell to think up these combinations. These unconscious cells are given the ability to involve themselves in these combinations by the will of Allah. This is because **"...When He decides on something, He just says to it, 'Be!' and it is." (Surat al-Baqara:117)**

No other force in the heavens and on the earth save Allah is capable of ordering even a single feature of the trillions of cells. It becomes possible only by the will of Allah that a cell performs such mathematical operations as producing the most appropriate weapon to inactivate every enemy that has invaded the cell.

Brave Warriors: T cells

Some lymphocytes migrate to the thymus after they are manufactured in the bone marrow. The lymphocytes, which multiply and mature here, are called T cells. These cells mature to form two different types: killer and helper T cells. After a three-week education, T cells migrate to the spleen, lymph nodes, and intestinal tissues to wait for the time of their mission.

The T cell Pathway

In comparison to B cells, T cells must go through a much more complicated course to be ready to commence their mission. Just like B cells, they, too, are simple cells in the beginning. These simple cells go through a series of difficult tests to become a T cell.

Lymphoid progenitor cell

Lymphoblast

Monoblast

Lymphocyte

In lymph tissue

Promonocyte

B cell lymphocyte

In blood

T- cell lymphocyte

Monocyte

In the first test, it is checked whether the cell can recognize the enemy or not. The cells recognizes the enemy with the assistance of "MHC"(Major Histocompatibility Complex) located on the surface of the enemy, which is a molecule that subjects the antigen to a series of chemical processes and presents it to the T cells.

Eventually, only those cells that are able to identify the enemy can survive. The others are not tolerated and they are immediately destroyed.

The recognition of enemy cells alone does not ensure the survival of T cells. These cells must also have a very good knowledge of the harmless substances and the regular tissues of the human body so to as prevent unnecessary conflict, which will eventually harm the body.

The white cells made in the lymph system tissue develop into lymphocytes (B cells and T cells) or monocytes. Lymphocytes are key players in immune responses. Mmonocytes can transform into large phagocytic (engulfing) cells called macrophages.

What is the MHC (Major Histocompatibility Complex) Molecule?

MHC is a molecule specially created to help the T cells in recognizing the enemy. They subject the antigen to a series of chemical processes and present it to the T cells. With the aid of MHC molecules, virus particles, cancer cell molecules, and even particles belonging to the inner part of a bacterium can be detected.

There is a very important reason for the T cells to use MHC molecules. This helps them to penetrate host cells and locate camouflaged viruses. However, even the help of the MHC molecule is not sufficient for T cells to fulfill their function. T cells also need a helper cell. Called the APC (antigen-presenting cells) for the sake of brevity, these cells break antigens apart and grab a very important part from the antigen. This part contains the amino acid sequence that determines the antigen's identity. The T cell is activated when it receives this identity information from the APCs.

As we can see, there is a need for a superb sub-system for the defence system even to start a war. The absence of even a single component of this intelligence network, made up of many interconnected subunits, would render the system useless. Under these circumstances, it would be beyond reason to talk about coincidence in the formation of such an intelligence system. Entertaining such views would be verging on superstition.

There is wisdom at all levels of this system which has been flawlessly created by Allah. An example of this would be the performance of APC cells that bring the enemy to T cells. These cells are aware that T cells can recognize the enemy from its amino acid sequence. This is one of the thousands of pieces of evidence that both cells are created by the same power, that is, Allah.

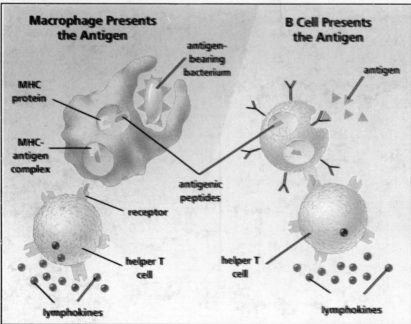

Macrophage Presents the Antigen

B Cell Presents the Antigen

antigen-bearing bacterium

antigen

MHC protein

MHC-antigen complex

antigenic peptides

receptor

helper T cell

helper T cell

lymphokines

lymphokines

Either a macrophage or a B cell presents an antigen to a helper T cell. To accomplish this, the antigen has to be digested to peptides that are combined with an MHC protein. The complex is presented to the T cell. In return, the helper T cell produces and secretes lymphokines that stimulate T cells and other immune cells.

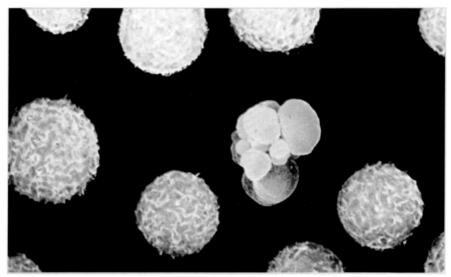

A cell destroying itself (middle). This programmed self-destruction is for the replacement of tissues or the elimination of damaged cells.

The T cell's Differentiation

According to the Order It Receives

The war has not yet ended for the T cells. Some T cells-to-be destroy themselves after receiving a specific signal from other cells.

There is very limited information on the signals that cause the cells to die a programmed death, to continue to live, or to mature and transform themselves. From a scientific point of view, this remains one of the unsolved mysteries of the defence system. Many similar cells in our body receive signals from somewhere, and start functioning upon this signal. How can these cells, which send signals to one another, be aware of the need to send a signal? Mahlon B. Hoagland brings up the same question in his book, *The Roots of Life*:

> *How do the cells know when to stop growing? What tells them that the organs of which they're a part are not just the right size?... What is the nature of the division stopping signal(s)? We don't know the answer and we continue to search for it.* [10]

Indeed, the mystery of the signaling between cells has not been solved yet.

A stem cell would normally be expected to divide to form two new cells bearing the same features. However, a switch hidden in one of the cells is turned on causing a sudden transformation in the cell. This new cell is the T cell that will fight for the human body. This leads us to ask the following question:

Why does a cell transform itself into a totally different cell?

Science has not answered this question yet. Science can answer the question of how the cell transforms itself, but it can never explain why the cell would want to become a fighter cell. Nor can it explain who programmed the cell to become a cell that defends the body when the need arises.

Only those who acknowledge the being of Allah can fully comprehend the answers to these questions.

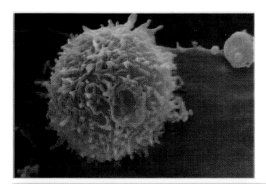

A T cell (left) can get orders to kill from a dendritic cell (bottom left, background) or a macrophage (bottom right).

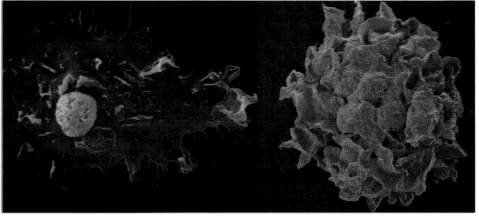

Types of T cells

T cells come in three groups: helper T cells, killer T cells, and suppressor T cells. Every T cell has a special MHC molecule enabling it to recognize the enemy.

Helper T cells

These cells can be regarded as the administrators of the system. In the initial stages of war, they decipher the properties of the foreigner cells absorbed by the macrophages and other antigen catcher cells. After they receive the due signal, they stimulate killer T and B cells to fight. This stimulation causes B cells to produce weapons called antibodies.

How do Helper-T cells start action?

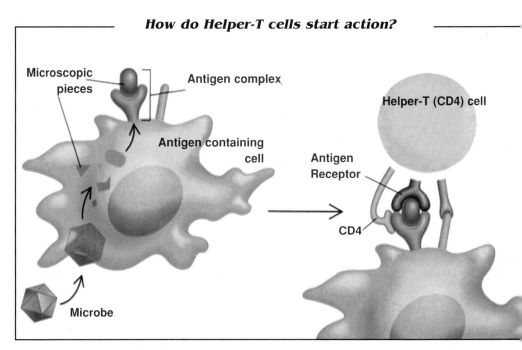

The picture illustrates how a cell breaks a microbe apart and presents it to the T cell. As the picture at the right indicates, the T cell will be activated only if its antigen receptor fits to the presented antigen, if the CD4 molecule adheres to the antigen complex, and if some other molecules (right) combine with each other. These safety mechanisms prevent a mature T cell from moounting an immune attack against its host.

Helper T cells secrete a molecule called lymphokine to stimulate other cells. This molecule somehow turns on a switch in other cells and starts off the war alarm.

The ability of the helper T cell to produce a molecule, which activates another cell, is a very important process.

First, the production of this molecule is related to an impending war strategy. It is obvious that the cells cannot make up this strategy themselves, nor can the strategy come about by sheer coincidence.

Developing a strategy would not be enough either. The molecule in the cell, which will switch on the production key in the other cell, should be synthesized accurately. For this, it has to be perfectly aware of the chemical structure of the opposite cell.

A mistake made in the production of this molecule alone would paralyze the defence system entirely. This is because an army without communication would be destroyed even before it launched its defence.

The existence of this molecule alone suffices to prove the absurdity of the theory of evolution. This is because the prerequisite of the system is the existence of this molecule right from the outset. If helper T cells failed to alert other cells with the help of this molecule, the human body would surrender to viruses.

Killer T cells

The killer T cells are the most efficient elements of the defence system. In previous chapters, we have studied how viruses are inactivated by proteins called antibodies. There are cases, however, when antibodies cannot reach out to a virus which has invaded a cell. On such occasions, killer T cells kill the sick cell which is invaded by the virus.

A closer examination of how killer T cells kill sick cells would reveal a great wisdom and an artistry in creation.

The killer T cells first have to distinguish between normal cells and those in which invaders hide. They deal with this problem with the help

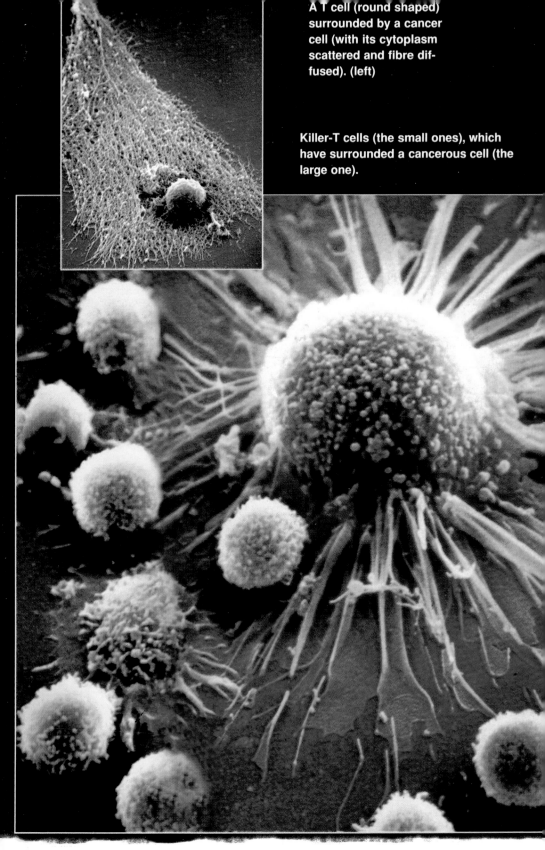

A T cell (round shaped) surrounded by a cancer cell (with its cytoplasm scattered and fibre diffused). (left)

Killer-T cells (the small ones), which have surrounded a cancerous cell (the large one).

of the innate system (MHC molecules) granted to them. When they locate the invaded cell, they secrete a chemical substance. This secretion sinks into the membrane of the cell forming a hole by lining up sideways in close formation. Following this, leaking starts in the cell which is full of pores, and the cell dies.

Killer T cells store this chemical weapon in granular form. This way, this chemical weapon is always kept ready for use. Scientists were amazed to discover the fact that the cell produces its own weapon by itself and stores it for future use. Even more amazing are the details in the mind-boggling way the cell uses this chemical weapon.

When an enemy approaches the host cell, these microgranules move to the tip of the cell in the direction of the enemy. Afterwards, they come in contact with the cell membrane, melt into it, and by extending towards the outside, they release the substance contained within them.

Natural Killer Cells: "NK"

These lymphocytes, which are produced in the bone marrow, are also available in the spleen, lymph node, and the thymus. Their most important functions are killing tumour cells and virus-carrier cells.

From time to time, invader cells take very sinister courses. They sometimes hide so well in body cells that neither antibodies nor T cells recognize the enemy. Everything seems usual from the outside. In such cases, the defence system somehow suspects an anomaly and "NK" cells rush to that region through the blood. Killer lymphocytes surround the cell and start to push the cell around. At that stage, the enemy cell is killed by a toxigenic substance injected inside it.

How these cells identify the enemy is yet another unanswered question about the defence system. The receptors that should be present on their surfaces to enable them to identify of the target cells have not yet been discovered. Therefore, the mechanism they employ in identifying the enemy has not yet been clearly understood.

Despite all the technology at its disposal, mankind has still not been able to solve the details of the system these cells use to identify the enemy. Perhaps future technological advances will throw light on this system and this subject will no longer be a mystery. This, too, would be a piece of evidence proving the perfection of the current system, and what an intricate plan is involved in its creation.

Blood Cells

- **Thrombocytes:** The coagulation of blood is considered an ordinary event, which is largely ignored by people. However, if the perfect system which makes this possible had not existed, human beings would experience significant risks and even bleed to death from the slightest injuries. The thrombocyte, which is one of the blood cells produced in the bone marrow, serves this function. It also includes a substance called serotonin that plays an important role in allergic reactions.

- **Eosinophil:** These blood cells have the ability to perform phagocytosis, i.e. destroy (phagocytose) any foreign cells entering the body.

- **Basophil:** A big, rough and single-nucleus blood cell which is found in small quantities in the blood, and abundantly in the dermal, splenic and intestinal connective tissues.

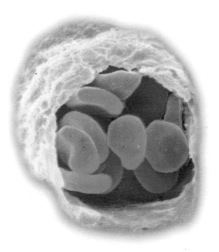

- **Neutrophils:** With an antibacterial quality, these blood cells protect the organism against foreign materials. In addition, they help the defence system with their phagocytosis capabilities.

Antigen Presenting Cells: "APC"

The duty of these cells is to present the antigen (enemy) to the T cells. Why a cell would serve such a function

Blood cells

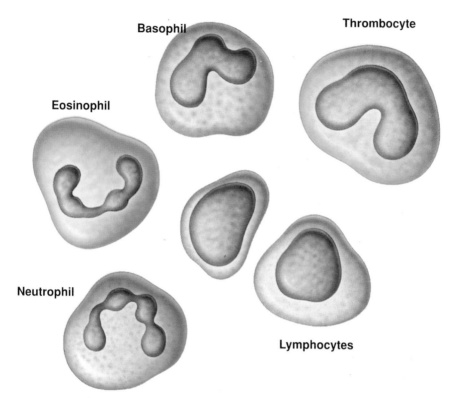

Above are the pictures of blood cells.

— an important responsibility — definitely needs further consideration. It knows that the T cells defend the human body, identify the enemy and present the enemy it captures to the T cells for them to provide intelligence about it.

Why would the cell do this? According to the theory of evolution, this cell should be concerned only about its own well-being. However, it serves the system, although it receives no benefit from it.

What is even more interesting is that the APC are very well aware of the requirements of the T cells. Based on this, the APC will break down the enemy cell and present to the T cell only the amino acid sequence. This

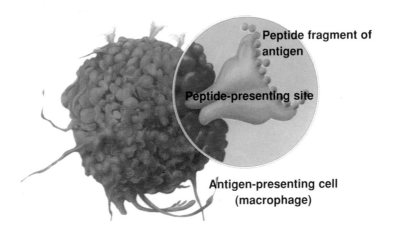

Peptide fragment of
antigen

Peptide-presenting site

Antigen-presenting cell
(macrophage)

Examples of APCs are macrophages. They do this by taking the foreign material into a cavity in their cytoplasm - the part of the cell outside the nucleus - and adding digestive chemicals to them. These chemicals break the bacteria into fragments of the proteins from which they are made, fragments that are now harmless, but which can also be utilized.

means that the APC is even aware that the T cell will extract the required information from this sequence.

At this point, it would be useful to recall one thing: We mentioned actions such as "knowing", "calculating", "thinking", "serving". Unquestionably, those actions require a certain consciousness. It is virtually impossible for a being with no consciousness or will to perform these actions. Yet, here we are talking about these abilities as being inherent in these minuscule entities: common, tiny, unconscious cells. Therefore, who gives this consciousness, ability, and a glorious system to these cells?

The answer to this question is very evident. It is Allah Who creates the APC and the T cell, as well as all other cells in the body, in a harmonious way to serve in the same system.

STEP BY STEP TO ALL-OUT WAR

Until now, we have discussed the general structure of the defence system, its organs, cells, and enemies. In this chapter, we will explore the deadly warfare between our defence system and enemy cells, and the wonderful defence our body mounts.

The brave battle fought by of our defence system is comprised of three important stages:

1. Identification of the enemy, first action.
2. The attack of the real army, all-out war.
3. Retreat to a normal state.

The defence system has to clearly identify the enemy before it starts the fight. This is because each engagement differs from the other depending on the type of enemy. Moreover, if this piece of intelligence is not properly handed on, our defence system may inadvertently attack the body's own cells.

The phagocytes, known as the scavenger cells of the defence system, take the first action. They fight hand-to-hand with the enemy. They are just like infantrymen who fight with bayonets against enemy units.

Sometimes, phagocytes cannot catch up with the increasing numbers of the enemy, at which point big phagocytic cells, macrophages cut in. We can liken the macrophage to cavalrymen cleaving their way through the middle of the foe. At the same time, macrophages secrete a fluid, which

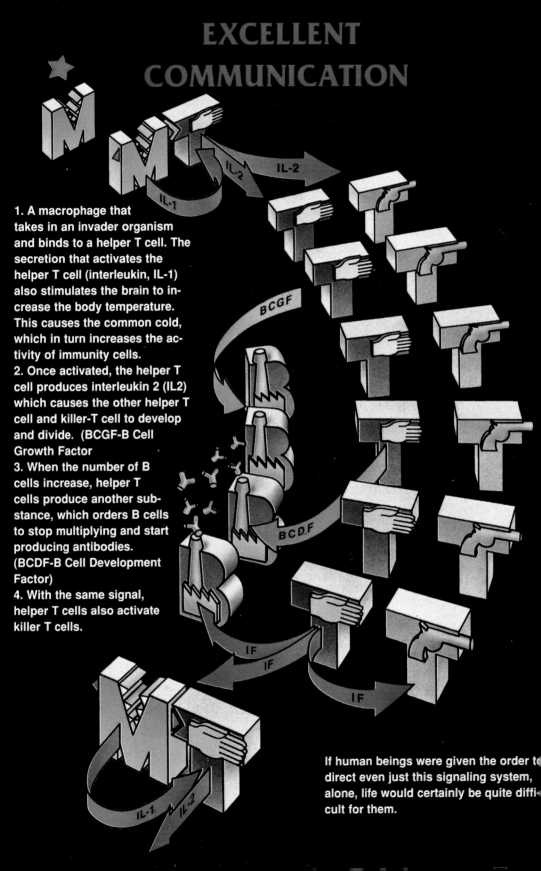

EXCELLENT COMMUNICATION

IL-2

IL-2

IL-1

BCGF

BCDF

IF

IF

IF

IL-1

IL-2

1. A macrophage that takes in an invader organism and binds to a helper T cell. The secretion that activates the helper T cell (interleukin, IL-1) also stimulates the brain to increase the body temperature. This causes the common cold, which in turn increases the activity of immunity cells.

2. Once activated, the helper T cell produces interleukin 2 (IL2) which causes the other helper T cell and killer-T cell to develop and divide. (BCGF-B Cell Growth Factor

3. When the number of B cells increase, helper T cells produce another substance, which orders B cells to stop multiplying and start producing antibodies. (BCDF-B Cell Development Factor)

4. With the same signal, helper T cells also activate killer T cells.

If human beings were given the order to direct even just this signaling system, alone, life would certainly be quite difficult for them.

sets off a general alarm in the body to increase the body temperature.

Macrophages have yet another important characteristic. When a macrophage cell captures and engulfs a virus, it tears off a special portion of the virus, which it carries on itself like a flag. This serves as a sign for the other elements of the defence system as well as an item of information.

Once the gathered intelligence is forwarded to the helper T cells, by the help of which they identify the enemy, their first task is to immediately alert the killer T cells, stimulating them to multiply. Within a short period, the stimulated killer T cells will become a formidable army. This is not the only function of the helper T cells. They also ensure that more phagocytes arrive at the battlefront while they transfer the gathered intelligence relating to the enemy to the spleen and lymph nodes.

Once the lymph nodes receive this information, the B cells, which have been waiting for their turn, are activated. (The B cells are manufactured in the bone marrow and then migrate to the lymph nodes to wait for their turn to be of service).

The activated B cells go through a number of stages. Every stimulated B cell begins to multiply. The multiplication process continues until thousands of identical cells are formed. Then, the B cells, which are ready for war, start to divide and are transformed into plasma cells. Plasma cells also secrete antibodies, which will be used as weapons during the fight with the enemy. As stated in earlier chapters, B cells are capable of producing thousands of antibodies in a second. These weapons are very handy. They are capable enough to bind to the enemy first, and then to destroy the biological structure of the enemy (antigen).

If the virus penetrates the cell, the antibodies cannot capture the virus. At this point, the killer T cells come into play again and, by identifying the viruses in the cell with the help of MHC molecules, they kill the cell.

However, if the virus has been successfully camouflaged, escaping even the notice of killer T cells, then "natural killer cells", briefly called NKs, swing into action. These cells destroy the cells which host viruses in them, and which are imperceptible to other cells.

CELL WARS

The Virus

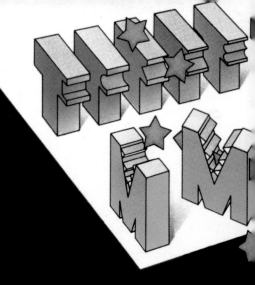

The Macrophage

The Helper T cell

The Killer T cell

The B Cell

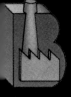

The Antibody

The Suppressor T cell

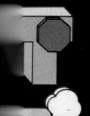

The Memory Cell

1 *THE WAR BEGINS*

As viruses start to invade the body, some will be captured by the antigens with the assistance of the macrophages and subsequently destroyed. Some of millions of T helper cells travelling in the circulatory system have the ability to "read" this specific antigen. These particular T cells become active when they bind to the macrophages.

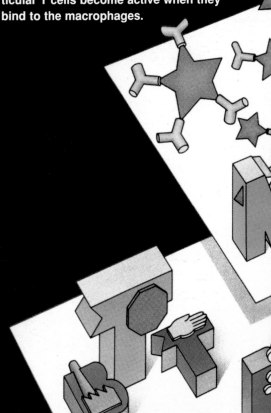

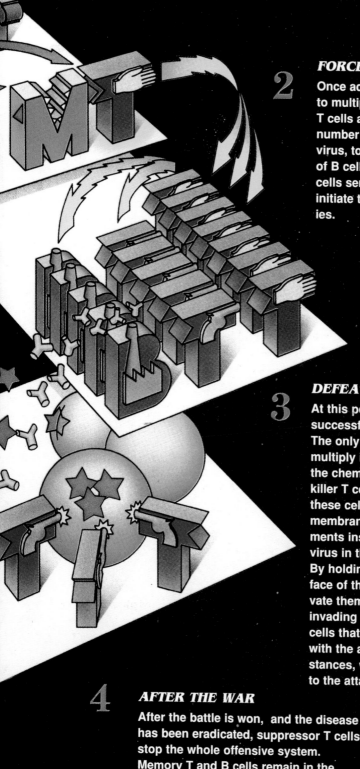

FORCES MULTIPLY

2 Once activated, helper T cells begin to multiply. They then warn the killer T cells and B cells, which are few in number and sensitive to the enemy virus, to multiply. When the number of B cells increases, the helper T cells send them a type of signal to initiate the manufacturing of antibodies.

DEFEATING THE INFECTION

3 At this point, some viruses have successfully penetrated the cells. The only place where viruses can multiply is in the body cells. With the chemical materials they secrete, killer T cells cause the death of these cells by drilling through their membranes, and removing the elements inside. Thus they prevent the virus in the cell from reproducing. By holding directly on to the surface of the virus, antibodies inactivate them and prevent them from invading other cells. In conclusion, cells that are infected are destroyed with the aid of chemical substances, which were prepared prior to the attack.

AFTER THE WAR

4 After the battle is won, and the disease has been eradicated, suppressor T cells stop the whole offensive system. Memory T and B cells remain in the blood and lymphatic system in order to become immediately activated in case a virus of the same type is met.

After the victory is won, suppressor T cells stop the war. Although the war is over, it is never to be forgotten. Memory cells have stored the enemy in their memory. Staying in the body for years, these cells help the defence to be faster and more effective if the same enemy is encountered again.

The heroes of this war have not received any military training.

The heroes of this war are not human beings able to reason.

The heroes of this war are cells so minuscule as to hardly cover a full stop when they come together in millions.

Moreover, this amazing army does not engage in fighting alone. It manufactures all the weapons it will use during the war; it makes all war plans and strategies itself, and cleans up the battleground after the war. If all these processes were left in the control of man, and not cells, would we ever be able to handle such a feat of organization?

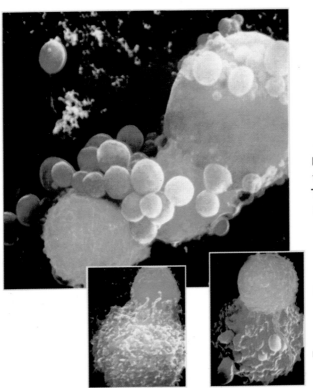

Millions of lymphocytes circulating within our bloodstream are charged with the responsibility of destroying harmful organisms contained in the human body. In these pictures, you can see a killer T cell (orange) attacking a cancer cell. The T cell destroys the protective membrane of the cancer cell with the help of its caustic enzymes and destroys the cell. At the end of the attack the only thing that remains is the large, round, almost naked nucleus of the cancer cell. (large picture)

What if the War in the Body Were Left in the Control of Humans Beings

People do not immediately realize that microbes or viruses are invading their bodies. Only when the symptoms of their illness surface do humans become aware of them. This is proof that a virus, a bacterium, or a similar micro-organism has long ago settled within their body. This means that the primary intervention has resulted in failure. Such unchecked conditions could cause the disease to progress considerably, resulting in irremediable dispositions. Even if the person has been infected with a curable and relatively simple disease, delayed response may result in a serious crisis, or even death.

Now, let us imagine that the coordination and control of the elements of the defence system and the ensuing strategies to be developed and implemented, the overseeing of the war itself were all left to human beings. What sort of difficulties would we confront?

Let us assume that the initial symptoms were effectively diagnosed. When foreign cells enter the human body, immediately the warrior cells must be manufactured and then sent to the area of conflict. The B cells must immediately commence the production of the weapon (antibody). How are we to determine the type and location of these foreign cells? This is a significant point, as future treatment depends on this initial stage. To do this, the only solution for the person would be to have a medical check-up which covered all the organs of his body down to every drop of his blood at the slightest suspicion of invaders having entered the body. Otherwise, it would be impossible to determine the type and location of the antigens. The long time needed for such a process would undoubtedly cause a serious delay in timely intervention. It is evident how troublesome and distressful life would be for people if they had to go to the doctor's to undergo such a check-up on the merest hint of infection.

Let us suppose that timely intervention was possible and the type and location of antigens could be identified precisely. Depending on the type of the enemy, first the phagocytes have to be activated. How can phagocytes be directed to rush to the exact location? What kind of a message would help them to locate the enemy easily? Let us suppose that the impossible became the possible. Then comes the time to learn whether the phagocytes have won the war or not. Depending on the result, either the macrophages will be launched or the war will be stopped. No doubt, the only possible solution lies with visiting the doctor again and having a thorough check-up. If the war has not been won, the secondary forces, that is, the macrophages, must be sent to the area of conflict. Meanwhile, the time spent on the check-up would work against us. Without losing any time, the macrophages have to tear a piece off the enemy and warn the helper T cells. The helper T cells will in turn warn the killer T cells, thus initiating another struggle. These cells, too, must be checked on as to whether they are successful or not — for which, again, a doctor's help is needed — and then the NK cells must be called in for assistance. After a final examination, it will be determined if the defence system has been effective in defeating the infection.

If man were asked to control only his defence system and nothing else, he would have to be involved in such a complicated and difficult process. Even a simple common cold would require him to go to the doctor's many times over, follow up the recovery course of the cells with extremely advanced medical equipment, and direct them as necessary. Even the slightest delay or a problem in the course of the process would cause the illness to be further aggravated.

What if man were asked to form these cells, make them recognize the enemy and manufacture the appropriate antibodies, then teach and organize all the processes they would perform ... Unquestionably, such a life would be far more troublesome and distressful than the aforementioned model. It would literally be impossible.

Allah has taken the burden of this process away from humans, creating a faultless system to work in the most immaculate and independent manner ever imaginable. Just like everything else in the universe, our defence system, too, has obeyed its purpose of creation to become an indispensable, critical element of life:

Hearkening to its Lord as it is bound to do...(Surat al-Inshiqaq: 2)

Tolerance

We have explored in previous chapters how the defence system distinguishes between friendly and hostile cells with the help of the receptors. However, the building blocks of some hostile cells are almost identical to those of certain tissues in the human body. This represents a significant problem for the defence system, which might conceivably attack some of its own tissues accidentally.

Under normal conditions, though, such a response never happens in a healthy human body. The defence system never attacks a molecule, cell, or tissue of its own. In medical terms this phenomenon is referred to as "tolerance".

This constitutes an extremely important miracle. We can clearly see that the defence system is fully capable of differentiating between thousands of proteins. For example, the defence system must distinguish the haemoglobin found in blood from the insulin secreted by the pancreas and from the vitreous humour contained in the eye, and indeed, from everything else in the human system. The defence system knows that while it fights a merciless war against foreign molecules, it must not harm any tissues belonging to the human body.

For many years, researchers have tried to understand how the defence system has learned to be tolerant towards its own tissues. Yet, details concerning why the most important lymphocytes, namely, the T and B cells, do not attack the human body have only been revealed in the last 20 years. The tolerance process, only a small portion of which mankind has been able to discover as the result of years long research, has been in operation since the human being came into existence.

How then has the defence system possessed the ability to distinguish the various different structures from each other? Can this be the result of unconscious coincidences as the theory of evolution suggests? It is certainly impossible for structures made up of unconscious atoms to coincidentally acquire this selection ability that requires such consciousness, information and intelligence.

When specially designed structures of lymphocytes enabling them to make the right choise is investigated, it will be understood how illogical and unreasonable the claim of evolutionists is.

A defence cell developed within the bone marrow or the thymus would be killed or inactivated if it reacted to the products of the body. A mature lymphocyte faces the same consequence in case it attacks the body's own products. That is to say that any element of the defence system likely to harm the body is either killed or forced to commit suicide obeying the command it receives.

However, if a T cell is confronted by another body cell, it does not at-

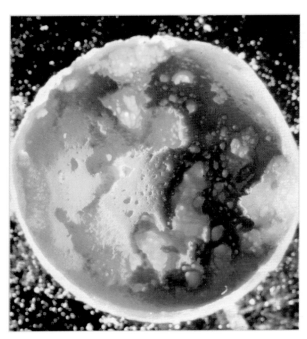

Elements of the defence system can harm themselves if they are unable to distinguish between friendly and enemy cells. Here you can see the organism attacking its own cell as if it were an enemy.

tack but rather inactivates itself. Similarly, if there is any substance in the body that carries antigen properties which should not, however, be destroyed, the human body does not produce any antibodies and so does not attack it.

If we consider the fact that our body contains around 1 trillion lymphocytes, we can appreciate the miraculous discipline required to ensure that these cells only target enemy cells and spare friendly cells.

The Protected Barrier

In essence, the embryo in a mother's womb should normally be considered foreign matter by the host human body. Subsequently, when the embryo is first formed, the body would immediately instigate a struggle against it. The defence system would not allow such an 'enemy' to develop. However, despite this negative scenario, the embryo is not as vulnerable as we might assume. After it is formed, it succeeds in fully developing over an extended period of 9 months, completely protected against the intended attacks of the antibodies.

How then is this achieved?

There is a barrier surrounding the embryo specially created to absorb only the nutrients in the blood. This barrier helps the embryo to take up the necessary nutrients for its development, while isolating it from the destructive effect of antibodies.

Otherwise, the antibodies would immediately attack the embryo (considered as a foreign substance) and destroy it. The isolation of the embryo from the antibodies with such a special protection is one of the most perfect examples of creation in the mother's womb.

Neither mutation, nor natural selection nor any other so-called evolutionary mechanism could have incorporated such perfect creation in the evolution tale. The miracle of creation is self-evident. In the Qur'an, Allah states that He placed the embryo in a secure repository:

Did We not create you from a base fluid. then place it in a secure

repository for a recognised term? It is We who determine. What an excellent Determiner! (Surat al-Mursalat: 20-23)

There are occasions when these cells fail to fulfill their functions. However, it should never be forgotten that if Allah had willed, this would not happen either. Such disorders are created for a hidden cause for people to clearly comprehend how temporary and incomplete the life of this world actually is. Were it not for the existence of a variety of diseases and illnesses, humans would be likely to forget how helpless they were against Allah Who created them. They might fail to remember that no matter how advanced technology is, their recovery, as well as their life, depend on the will of Allah alone. They may continue to live as if they will remain in good health forever, as if they will never meet death and be called to account for their actions in the presence of Allah on the Day of Judgment. They may live on without reflecting on the plight of those who are sick, deprived and oppressed. Therefore, they may fail to appreciate that their health is a blessing from Allah and that they should live their lives in the most favorable and productive way. People of this sort, however, hardly ever accept these facts, which we have listed above. Illnesses make people accept them in a flash. It is not until then that people start to think about things that never occurred to them before, such as their helplessness and incapacity against the power of Allah, the fact that technology, which developed by the will of Allah, can again only be of any use by His will; they think of those people in need, of death, and depending on their illness, even the stage beyond death. Only then do people appreciate their health. Furthermore, they witness the undependability of the life of this world, to which they were blindly devoted and committed with all their existence; this causes them to re-assess whether they have worked enough for the hereafter, their true abode.

Indeed, our true abode is not this world, but the hereafter. Life in the hereafter is not limited by years, nor is its quality dictated by such basic needs as sleeping, feeding, or cleaning, or by negative factors such as diseases. The endless blessings in heaven are stated in the following verse of the Qur'an:

They will remain there timelessly, for ever, among everything their selves desire. (Surat al-Anbiya: 102)

It is a pity that the majority of people do not appreciate their health, or think of the fleeting nature of the life of this world. And only if they fall ill do they pray to Allah. When, however, they are restored to health and return to their daily lives, they forget everything. In the Qur'an, Allah draws attention to this characteristic of humans:

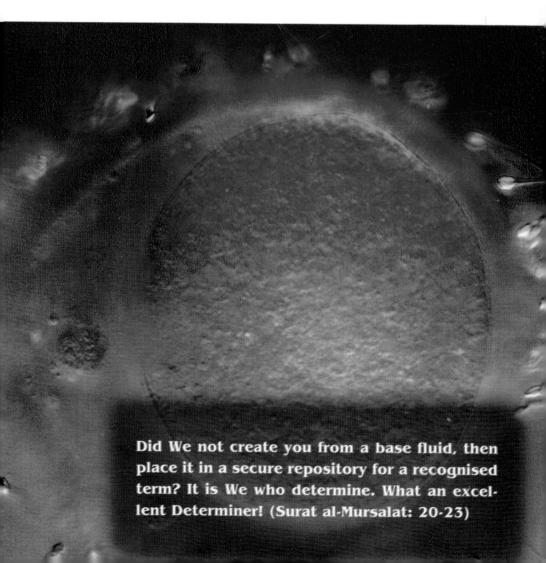

Did We not create you from a base fluid, then place it in a secure repository for a recognised term? It is We who determine. What an excellent Determiner! (Surat al-Mursalat: 20-23)

When harm touches people they call on their Lord, repenting to Him. But then, when He gives them a taste of His mercy, a group of them immediately associate others with their Lord (Surat ar-Rum: 33)

Allah, Who knows the truth of things (al-Khabir), created thousands of types of diseases, all of which lie in store for human beings. There is no guarantee that one of them, maybe the most dangerous one, will not infect you. Every miraculous organ and system in our body is apt to wear down and fail to operate. As we have stated earlier, if Allah had willed it so, none of this would happen and no problems would occur in any of our organs and systems. It is obvious that there is a message delivered to human beings in all these happenings, that is the temporary nature of the life of this world...

THE ENEMIES
OF THE SYSTEM

In most general terms, cancer can be characterized as uncontrolled cell replication. Regardless of its type, cancer initially develops in a normal, healthy cell and shares the basic characteristics of this normal cell, at least in its early developmental stages. However, these cells tend to lose some of their abilities. One such important ability is that of reacting to the messages delivered by their surrounding or their own organisms that regulate cell replication. When such a disorder occurs, the cell can no longer control its replication and the growth of tissues. This process, known as "continuous dividing," is genetically transferred to new cells resulting in the spread of tumours, which in turn invade the neighbouring tissues. These decomposed cells eat up the nutrients of other cells, consuming the vital amino acid supply. Cancer cells eventually shut down the passages within the human body with their expanding volume. They accumulate in various organs such as the brain, lungs, liver, and kidneys, surrounding the healthy and normal cells of these organs and preventing their normal functioning, eventually posing a serious threat to human life.

Normal cells replicate only when they receive a command from neighbouring cells. This is a safety measure within the organism. However, cancer cells do not respond to this mechanism and refuse any control over their replication system. The type of cancer described so far does not create any problem for the defence system. A strong body with an effect-ive defence system is capable of struggling with the increasingly expand-ing cancerous cells multiplying in number, and of even defeating the dis-ease. The main problem arises when cancer cells pierce their own mem-branes with the help of an enzyme (pac-man enzyme), and mix in the cir-culatory system (the conveyor network) of the body by penetrating the lymphatic fluid, and eventually reaching distant tissues and cells.

The current scenario is quite negative. Cells that used to work col-lectively in providing humans with the gifts of seeing, hearing, breathing, and living suddenly grow recalcitrant, not obeying the "stop" command they receive from neighbouring cells. As they continue replicating, they carry out a destruction process at full blast which leads to the total death of the body.

If we compare the human body to a country and the human defence system to a powerful, fully equipped army, the cancer cells emerge as the rebels of this country. This mutinous community grows in number daily, continuing their demolition of the current structure. But the army of this country is not at all pregnable.

The macrophages, the front line warriors of the defence system, sur-round the invader when they encounter it and destroy the cancer cells with the help of a protein they specially produce. In addition, the T cells, the strong and intelligent warriors of the defence system and their excep-tional weapons (antibodies) kill the cancer cells that have begun to fuse in

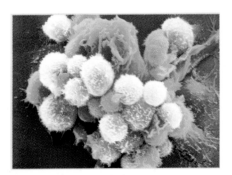 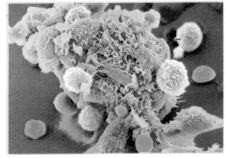

A war between the cancer cell (pink) and lymphocytes (yellow)

the body and lymphatic fluids by piercing the cell membrane. The struggle will continue even as the cancer spreads. As the cancer cells develop further, the defence cells help to inhibit the progress of the disease, resulting in remission.

One of the systems within human cells which prevent the spread of cancer cells is "apoptosis", which causes the suicide of the cell. Apoptosis is seen when the DNA of the cell is damaged, or a tumour develops, or the effectiveness of the P53 gene — also known as the "cancer preventing gene" — lessens. Though apoptosis may appear to be a very negative event, it is actually highly important, as it blocks such vital disorders and prevents the disease from passing on to the next generation. When compared to the potential danger imposed by the cancer cells, which are likely to damage the entire human body, the loss of a single cell is much more acceptable. Cells within the human body that realize (!) that there is a dis-

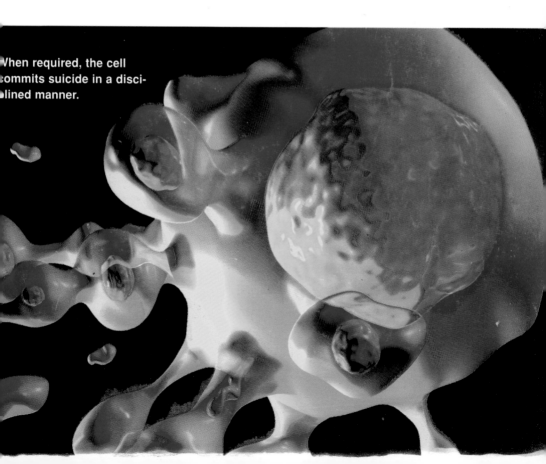

When required, the cell commits suicide in a disciplined manner.

order in their own structure threatening the human body instigate their own demise to prolong human life.

The cancer takes on a life-threatening form when these decomposed cells overcome this suicide system. In this case, a second defence mechanism is activated to avoid uncontrolled multiplying of these cells. If they succeed in surpassing this barrier, too, they then encounter a further stage known as the "the term of crisis". At this stage, the cells, which have successfully escaped from the previous security systems, are killed en masse. Among these cells, one cell, however, succeeds in overcoming the "crisis". This "rebellious" cancer cell will transfer its rebellious nature to its descendants, which will multiply in great numbers. The cancerous patient must now fight an intensive struggle with cancer.

Is it only the uncontrolled, independent and continuously multiplying nature of the cancer cell that brings victory to it? Other reasons lie behind this success.

Cells carry a type of inscription system on their surface which positions them in the body. This inscription system is decipherable by all the cells within the human body, helping each cell to know exactly where it belongs and preventing it from occupying another's place. This system ensures the integrity of the tissues. Cells, which are aware of their position, neither go anywhere else, nor let any other cell occupy their place, thus ensuring the maintenance of the body in a healthy state. Cells that are not located at a certain site or those located at an inappropriate site will eventually commit suicide. However, with the help of this system, the suicide process is totally eliminated, as the cells are not allowed to be dislocated or located in an inappropriate site. This process is not as simple as it may seem. In order to maintain the effective functioning of this system, each cell has to identify its own position whilst respecting the locations of other cells, and being mindful not to invade their sites. These procedures are taught to them by various mediator molecules which enable these cells to maintain their respective places. However, there are occasions when these mediator molecules are absent or unable to fulfil this duty.

This provides the cancer cells with an advantage. When inhibitory molecules are not present in the environment, cancer cells spread more rapidly. Besides, cancer cells are not required to anchor themselves to any specific site. They undermine the rules by living independently and without settling in any place.

Erythrocytes are exceptional cells that do not possess a stationary site within the human body. They pierce the membranes of other cells and tissues and tear down the obstacles with the aid of a special enzyme called "metallo-proteinase". They are therefore able to visit any part of the human body at will. The defence cells use this enzyme to reach out to the enemy cells, while cancer cells use them for an entirely different purpose. Their main goal is to attack healthy cells and invade them.

The skills of the cancer cells are not limited to these pursuits; they are also capable of playing other 'games' against the defence cells. Odd as it may sound, we are not talking about talented actors but rather cancer cells, which play games against their opponents. Before attempting to explain these unbelievably clever games, let us review what we have explained so far.

Isn't it extraordinary that our army of defence sets up progressive barriers against the enemy? This organization we call an "army" is made up of cells which can only be viewed under an advanced electron micro-

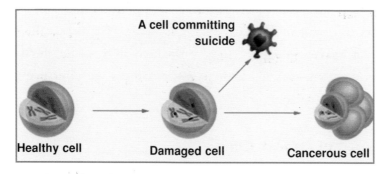

The process by which healthy cells transform into cancer cells. A normal cell as seen at the left either commits suicide or transforms into a cancer cell as it undergoes various genetic mutations.

scope. Their ability to protect and guard their sites, their willingness to lay down their own lives to save the life of the human body they belong to, their unyielding commitment to continue their struggle, are not the products of coincidence. Undoubtedly, we can see a very conscious and well-organized form of functioning in defence cells.

What would happen if such a difficult mission were handed to a trillion highly educated humans beings? Would the success rate be as impressive? Would it be possible for them to enforce their will on the crowd despite the existence of strict disciplinary rules and obligatory measures? If a few of these individuals forgot the formula of the antibodies they were supposed to manufacture, or neglected to manufacture them, or refused to commit suicide when necessary, would all of these stages function regularly? Would the struggle end with victory? Could an army of billions of individuals continue its struggle without any mistake? Are there, by any chance, any brave and skilled commanders or managers who would be willing to undertake the responsibility of keeping these billions under control? However, our defence cells do not need any commanders or managers. Their system operates in a very regulated manner, without any inhibitions or difficulties. There is no anarchy or confusion during the process. The reason for this perfection and extremely effective functioning is Allah, Who established this system down to its minute details and inspired the elements of this system to fulfill their responsibilities. In the 5th verse of Surat al-Sajda, it is stated: **"He directs the whole affair from heaven to earth."**. In accordance with this rule, the defence cells continue their struggle without rest or duress with this inspiration given to them by Allah.

Games of Cancer Cells

It must not be forgotten that cancer cells are original body cells that carry the molecular character of the human being. In consequence, it is difficult for the defence cells to identify cancer cells. Furthermore, cancer cells manage to win over some antibodies by a method undiscovered to date.

As we have mentioned, antibodies are a type of protein that stops the activities of enemy cells. However, for some unknown reason, cancer cells are adversely affected by the antibodies. Instead of stopping, their activities increase, resulting in the rapid and forceful spreading of the tumour.

Antibodies, which bind themselves on to the surface of the cancer cell, "collaborate" with the cancer cell in a sense. Other antibodies do not touch a cancer cell having an antibody attached to it. Hence, the cancer cell is perfectly camouflaged.

Collaboration between antibodies and cancer cells can reach even broader dimensions. There are also occasions where cancer cells combine with antibodies to form "pseudo supressor T cells". These pseudo suppressor T cells misinform antibodies by relaying the message that there is "no danger". More sinister situations also develop whereby the cancer cells develop into "Pseudo Helper T cells" instead of the pseudo suppressor T cells. In such situations, the message is delivered to a bigger number of antibodies. There can be no more convenient environment possible for the development of cancer cells.

Additionally, cancer cells may sometimes spread "trap antigens" in order to protect themselves from a possible attack by the defence system. These tumours spread out such large amounts of antigens from their surface that the blood stream is inundated with them. These antigens, however, are fake and cause no harm to the human body. However, the antibodies are not aware of this and they respond without delay by instigating a war against them.

During this chaos, the real and dangerous cancer cells continue to function, going undisturbed and undiscovered by the enemy.

An Intelligent Enemy: AIDS

In the previous chapters we discussed viruses and explained the importance of their role in the life of humans. Among these viruses, the most

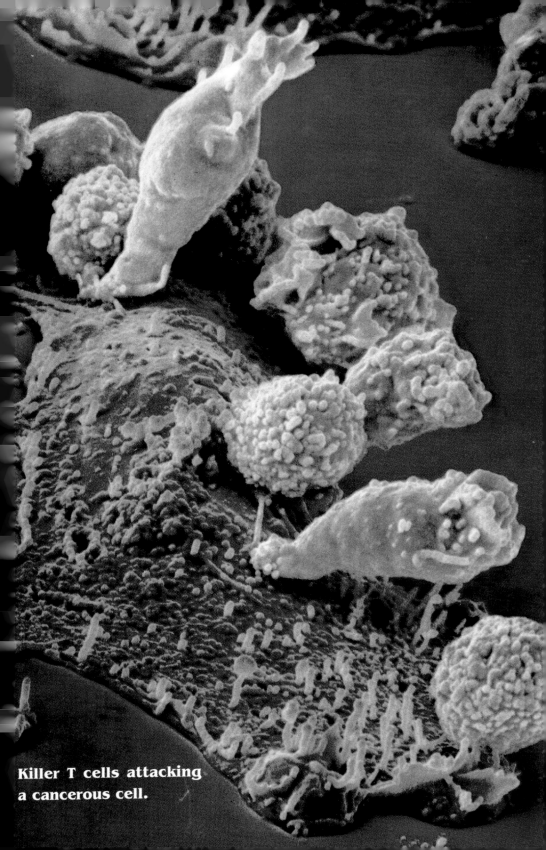

Killer T cells attacking a cancerous cell.

dangerous and harmful is the "HIV virus", which has preoccupied researchers for a long time and may well continue to do so for some time to come. Unlike other viruses, this micro organism totally inactivates the defence system. It is impossible for a human being with a malfunctioning defence system to survive.

The HIV virus causes irreversible damages to the human body by causing the defence system to collapse, making it vulnerable to all kinds of diseases, eventual-

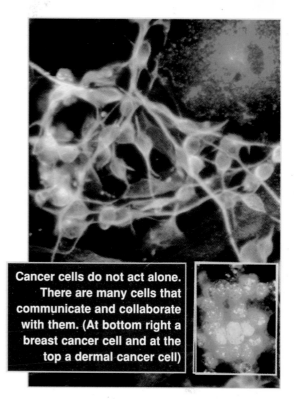

Cancer cells do not act alone. There are many cells that communicate and collaborate with them. (At bottom right a breast cancer cell and at the top a dermal cancer cell)

ly giving rise to various fatal conditions. It has occupied researchers for many years, resulting in a sense of desperation and hopelessness. *The Journal of Bilim ve Teknik (Science and Technology),* published in August 1993, made the following statement:

> *"The more we learn, the less certain we become." This statement is the most common answer to a public survey carried out among 150 of the most recognized researchers worldwide, studying AIDS. This was published in the weekly scientific journal Science. No one can make certain judgments based on the theses that have been advocated for years. Views, which were considered absolutely correct are now being pushed aside after they have been revealed to rely on shaky grounds. Inevitably, the end result is such that even long established theories about AIDS and its effective cause, the HIV virus are once again being reviewed and their validity being questioned.* [11]

With the passage of time, the issues have intensified rather than become resolved. To date there remains numerous unanswered questions, and the advent of new inventions has served only increase the number of these unanswered questions. AIDS still remains a mystery for mankind.

One of the most important facts known about the HIV virus is that it enters only some and not all the cells of human beings. Its main target is the helper T cells, which are the most effective elements of the defence system. This is a very important point. Among numerous types of cells, the virus chooses those cells of the defence system which are, in effect, the most beneficial for it and this instigates the destruction of the human body.

When T cells, the vital elements of the defence system, are seized, the defence system is deprived of its brain team, and is no longer able to recognize the enemy. This could be regarded as an ingenious war tactic. An army without any effective communication and intelligence systems would be considered to have lost its main strength.

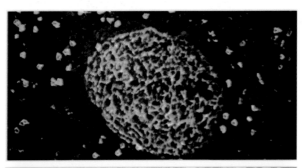

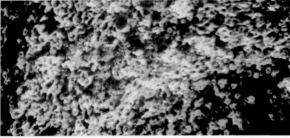

In the picture above you can see a healthy lymph node. The picture below shows a lymph node damaged by the AIDS virus.

Furthermore, the antibodies produced by the human body do not harm the AIDS virus. AIDS patients continue to produce antibodies, however, they are not as effective in the absence of the killer T cells.

One unanswered questions is: How does the HIV virus know exactly what target to focus on? By the time the AIDS virus understands that the T cells are regarded as the "brains" of the defence system, it will be destroyed by the existing system immediately upon entering the human body. However, it is impossible for the AIDS virus to conduct any form of intelligence surveillance prior to entering the human body. How then has the AIDS virus developed this strategy?

This is only the first of many amazing skills mastered by the AIDS virus.

At the second stage, the virus has to attach itself to the cells which it has set as a target for itself. This procedure is not at all difficult for the AIDS virus. In fact, it attaches to these cells as a key fits into its lock.

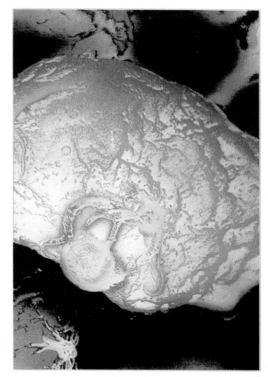

At the third stage, the HIV virus undergoes a series of miraculous processes, which will ensure its longevity.

The HIV virus is a retrovirus. This means that its genetic make-up contains solely RNA and no DNA. But a retrovirus needs DNA to remain alive. To provide this, it has recourse to

An AIDS virus (orange) attempting to enter a T cell by piercing the cell membrane.

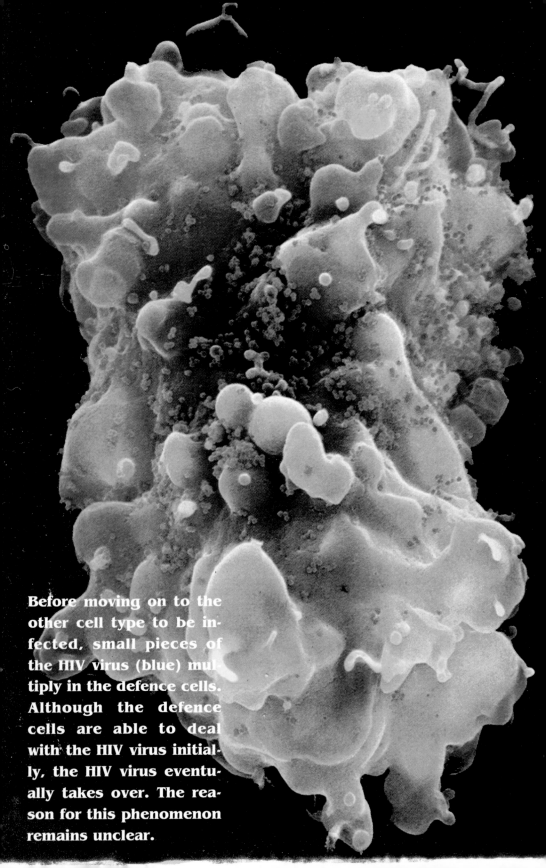

Before moving on to the other cell type to be infected, small pieces of the HIV virus (blue) multiply in the defence cells. Although the defence cells are able to deal with the HIV virus initially, the HIV virus eventually takes over. The reason for this phenomenon remains unclear.

a very interesting method: it uses the nucleic acids of its host cell and converts its RNA into DNA by means of an enzyme called "the reverse transcriptase", meaning it will reverse the process. Then it places this DNA in the DNA found in the nucleus of its host cell. The inheritance material of the virus has now become the inheritance material of the T cell. As the cell multiplies, so does the HIV virus. The cell starts to work as a factory for the virus. But invading a single cell does not satisfy the HIV virus. It will eventually attempt to seize the whole body.

Then the fourth stage comes. The initial HIV virus and others want to leave their host cells and invade other cells to facilitate their extraordinary proliferation. They do not expend much effort in doing so. Everything takes place at a natural pace. The membrane of the invaded T cells cannot tolerate the pressure of the multiplication process, and is riddled with holes, allowing the HIV viruses to get out of the cell to seek alternative hosts. As the HIV virus increases in number, it also kills its host T cell.

The successful HIV virus has now completely seized the human body. Unless mankind succeeds in discovering an effective cure to beat

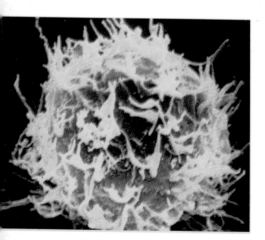 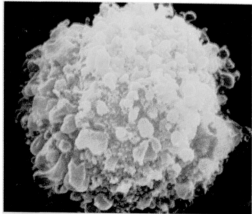

A healthy T cell.(left)
A T cell that has been destroyed by the enemy (the AIDS virus) and now possesses a round and softened profile.(right) These images are magnified more than 3000 times.

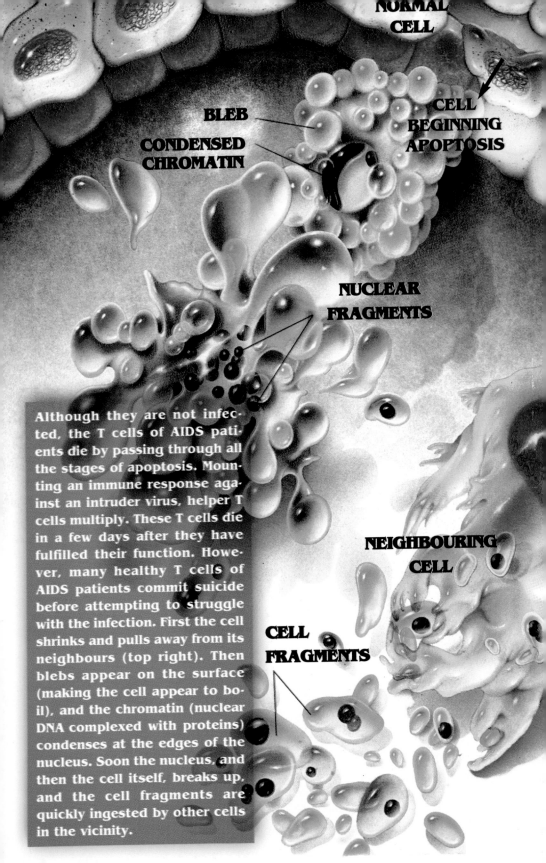

NORMAL
CELL

CELL
BEGINNING
APOPTOSIS

BLEB

CONDENSED
CHROMATIN

NUCLEAR
FRAGMENTS

NEIGHBOURING
CELL

CELL
FRAGMENTS

Although they are not infected, the T cells of AIDS patients die by passing through all the stages of apoptosis. Mounting an immune response against an intruder virus, helper T cells multiply. These T cells die in a few days after they have fulfilled their function. However, many healthy T cells of AIDS patients commit suicide before attempting to struggle with the infection. First the cell shrinks and pulls away from its neighbours (top right). Then blebs appear on the surface (making the cell appear to boil), and the chromatin (nuclear DNA complexed with proteins) condenses at the edges of the nucleus. Soon the nucleus, and then the cell itself, breaks up, and the cell fragments are quickly ingested by other cells in the vicinity.

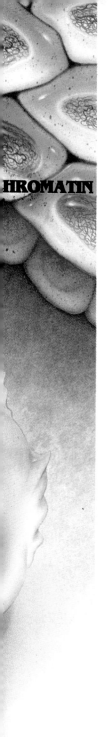

this virus, it will remain there. It is entirely at the discretion of the HIV virus either to lie dormant for many years, or instigate an immediate attack on the human body.

Why Has a Solution Not Yet Been Found?

After entering the human body, the HIV virus can produce up to ten billion viruses a day. The excessive number of viruses produced in one day is unmanageable, despite the technological advancements of the day. The HIV virus cannot be considered as a simple structure. What we have here is a micro-organism, so advanced and intelligent that it can duplicate millions of its own copies, possesses a plan to capture its host cell, and is able to cause the death of a huge human body.

In addition to the abilities of the HIV virus mentioned above, the HIV virus is also able to assume varying forms in an attempt to prevent its capture by the defence system. This makes the HIV virus immune to the effects of medications aimed at treating it today. Modern medicine has attacked the virus with a variety of medications at the same time and barely succeeded in dealing with the resistance of the virus. Although the virus is partially eradicated, the only positive outcome has been the prolonging of the patients' lives to a limited extent.

It is of great interest how a virus like the HIV virus can regenerate itself when faced with the danger of being eradicated. Scientists are left helpless in the presence of such skillful tactics.

These are not the only mind-boggling tactics used by the HIV virus. helper T cells circulating in the bloodstream swim along, interlocking with one another like the metallic projections of a zipper. The HIV leaps from one T cell to another to avoid contact with the antibodies in the blood stream. All this is done by a virus, which is only one micron in size, possesses no DNA and cannot even be qualified as a living creature. The extraordinary ability of the HIV virus to recognize the human body so well, develop advanced systems to overcome the human body, implement the necessary strategies without any errors and constantly modify itself to be protected from all kinds of weapons used by the body are all truly amazing. This is a very good example of how helpless mankind is rendered in the presence of a minute virus, which cannot be seen with the naked eye.

THE DEFENCE SYSTEM CANNOT HAVE BEEN FORMED BY EVOLUTION

According to statements of scientists, the defence system possesses an "irreducible complexity". This term refers to an intact system composed of several well-matched, interacting parts that contribute to the basic function, wherein the removal of any one of the parts causes the system to effectively cease functioning. As an example, let us think of the devices we would need if we were to send a fax:

- A facsimile device
- A telephone line
- A cable
- Paper.

If any one of these items is absent you cannot send a fax. Nothing from the above list must be missing. Besides, they must conform to exact specifications. For example, the length of the cable must be sufficient for the plug to reach the socket, otherwise the available items will be of no use. Similarly, although all elements of the defence system fulfill their functions perfectly, if there are a few components which malfunction, this would cause the body to lose the war. For example, if the tiny granules located within the T cells do not function properly, they cannot store toxins, which in turn cannot be transferred to the enemy, again resulting in the war being lost. Therefore, in a system where the enemy cannot finally be killed, important functions such as the formation of warrior cells, their training, the transmission of the necessary signals to appropriate locations by the cells at the right time, and the thousands of combinations needed by our genes to produce antibodies, or the storing of limitless information in the memory cells, would all be worthless. The system would simply not work. Similarly, the existence of the many and varied functions of the human body, which has an irreducible complexity, is equally useless in the absence of a defence system. If the defence system did not exist or failed to operate properly, no human being would be able to survive.

How then do evolutionists explain the formation of such a vital and complex system? Actually, they have no answers which can shed light on the subject. Their only assertion is based on the view that the defence system has developed through gradual evolutionary processes. They hold that the mechanisms that provide this gradual development are "natural selection" and "mutations".

But it is impossible for slight, successive coincidental modifications to produce such a complex system as the theory of evolution suggests. As emphasized before, the immune system would simply not function unless it existed with all its elements intact. To reiterate, a malfunctioning defence system would cause the human being to die within a short time.

The second point of the argument is the process of "Natural Selection". As we will explain in more detail in the chapter, "The Evolution Deceit", the process of "Natural Selection" refers to the transfer of advantageous qualities to subsequent generations.

There is a consensus among scientists that the concept of such a mechanism is far from being satisfactory in explaining complex systems. The renowned American specialist in biochemistry, Michael J. Behe, made the following statements with relation to natural selection in his book, *"Darwin's Black Box"*:

An irreducibly complex biological system, if there is such a thing, would be a powerful challenge to Darwinian evolution. Since natural selection can only choose systems that are already working, then if a biological system cannot be produced gradually it would have to arise as an integrated unit, at one fell swoop, for natural selection to have anything to react on. [12]

The founder of the theory of evolution, Charles Darwin, as well as many contemporary scientists, have confessed that the supposed mechanism of natural selection has no evolutionary power.

Charles Darwin states:

These difficulties and objections may be classed under the following heads:... Can we believe that natural selection could produce, on the one hand, an organ of trifling importance, such as the tail of a giraffe, which serves as a fly-flapper, and on the other hand, an organ so wonderful as the eye? [13]

One of the leading evolutionists of our day, professor of geology and paleoanthropology Dr Stephan Jay Gould states that natural selection can possess no evolutionary power:

But how do you get from nothing to such an elaborate something if evolution must proceed through a long sequence of intermediate stages, each favored by natural selection? You can't fly with 2 percent of a wing or gain much protection from an iota's similarity with a potentially concealing piece of vegetation. How, in other words, can natural selection explain these incipient stages of structures that can only be used (as we now observe them) in much more elaborated form? Mivart identified this problem as primary and it remains so today. [14]

Can the existence of such a complex system be explained, as suggested by Neo-Darwinists, in terms of "mutations"? Is it really possible for such an excellent system to form as a result of successive mutations?

As we know, mutations are decompositions and damage taking place in the genetic codes of living beings as a result of various external factors. All mutations damage the genetic information programmed in the DNA of a living being, without adding any new genetic information to it. Therefore, mutations do not possess any developmental or evolutionary faculty. Today, many evolutionists accept this reality, though reluctantly.

One of these evolutionists, John Endler, a geneticist from the University of California, comments:

> *Although much is known about mutation, it is still largely a "black box" relative to evolution. Novel biochemical functions seem to be rare in evolution, and the basis for their origin is virtually unknown.*[15]

The renowned French biologist Pierre P. Grassé also noted that the number of mutations would not change the result:

> *No matter how numerous they may be, mutations do not produce any kind of evolution.*[16]

It is clearly evident that the extraordinary properties and the mind-boggling abilities of these minute cells cannot be explained as mere coincidences or mutations; these are only evolutionists' fallacies, and are totally contradictory to science and logic. The highest human intelligence pales into insignificance when compared to the intelligence displayed by the cells.

There are thousands of similar extraordinary shows of intelligence in living creatures, which cannot be explained by the theory of evolution. In the face of these, many scientists, already plunged in doubt, are increasingly and day by day losing their confidence in the theory of evolution. They cannot help expressing their dissatisfaction at every opportunity.

Most researchers are well aware that evolutionist statements are nothing more than consolation and window-dressing. Klaus Dose, a well-known researcher in the field of molecular biology states:

> *More than 30 years of experimentation on the origin of life in the fields of chemical and molecular evolution have led to a better perception of the immensity of the problem of the origin of life on Earth rather than to its solution. At present all discussions on principal theories and experiments in the field either end in stalemate or in a confession of ignorance.* [17]

Even Darwin, the founder of the theory of evolution, experienced the same lack of confidence some 150 years ago:

> *When I think of the many cases of men who have studied one subject for years, and have persuaded themselves of the truth of the foolishest doctrines,*

I feel sometimes a little frightened, whether I may not be one of these mono-maniacs.[18]

It is quite evident that all these systems, just like everything else in the universe, are under the control of the Almighty Allah, the all-powerful and all-knowing. The inability of mankind to solve these mysteries is a sure sign that these issues are beyond man's grasp and are the product of greatly superior wisdom, that is, of Allah.

The answer to the questions which mankind has for centuries debated and deliberated upon, without being able to arrive at a logical conclusion, is extremely simple. The answer lies neither in coincidence, nor in natural selection nor in mutation. Not one of these is capable of forming life or maintaining its continuity.

The Qur'an provided the answers to all these questions 1400 years ago. Allah, the Lord of All the Worlds, has submitted our bodily cells as well as all that is in the universe to His Will:

Your Lord is Allah, Who created the heavens and the earth in six days and then settled Himself firmly on the Throne. He covers the day with the night, each pursuing the other urgently; and the sun and moon and stars are subservient to His command. Both creation and command belong to Him. Blessed be Allah, the Lord of All the Worlds. (Surat al-A'raf: 54)

CONCLUSION

I n this book, we explained the not so well known aspects of the army inside you, that is, your defence system. We have deliberately directed attention away from the complicated details of the extraordinary jobs the defence cells do to "how" the system operates. We searched for the answer to the question: "How can such minute cells which can be viewed only under an electron microscope produce such a complicated system as the defence system?" We delved further and examined how these cells, which make up the immune system were initially formed.

All cells of the immune system are initially normal cells, which go through different educative stages ending with a "Sufficiency Exam". Only those cells that are able to recognize enemy cells and do not conflict with other normal bodily cells are allowed to live. How and when was the first cell developed and who held the first "sufficiency exam"? Who has taught the cell what to do?

It is clearly unexpected that cells and associated organs can converse freely with each other, work in total agreement, make plans, and implement these plans efficiently. Do not forget that the topic of discussion here is numerous bodily organs and one trillion cells. It is impossible to imagine that one trillion people could be organized in such a perfect way and fulfill their duties without anything being skipped, forgotten, or confused, or any kind of chaos being caused in the mounting of such a defence, which is a supremely difficult task.

There is a definite reality, which must be accepted, and that is: cells, as well as everything in the universe without exception, from the smallest to the biggest, have been specially created by Allah Who possesses endless power, knowledge and wisdom.

...He created all things and He has knowledge of all things. (Surat al-An'am: 101)

This self-evident fact has been revealed in this book once again for all to see.

We mentioned that the unborn child in the mother's womb completes the missing components of its own defence system with the help of the antibodies received from its mother. However, if such possibilities were not available, or if these deficiencies continued following the child's birth, it would be impossible for the baby to survive. As we have repeatedly emphasized, given that mankind and countless other life forms are in existence today, this would mean that the defence system has been present from the very outset of life in its complete and fully functional form. It simply could not have been evolved in stages. It is a total impossibility that such an intensely complex system composed of interconnected, interdependent components, cells and elements could have been formed through minute coincidences over a period of millions of years.

Any person who suggests that everything has been formed through coincidences and refuses to accept that a "Creator" has created the entire universe, despite his awareness of the functioning of one or more than one miraculous system among numerous others continuously at work in his body, is also unaware that he has been mentioned in a clearly defined character type in the Qur'an some 1400 years ago. Allah has revealed in the Qur'an that such people are unable to comprehend even clear and open realities due to deficiencies in their perception and comprehension:

...They have hearts they do not understand with. They have eyes they do not see with. They have ears they do not hear with.... (Surat al-A'raf: 179)

Allah has again revealed that these people are actually aware of this situation;

They say, 'Our hearts are covered up against what you call us to and there is a heaviness in our ears. There is a screen between us and you...' (Surat al-Fussilat: 5)

Another group of disbelievers do see the realities presented, but proceed to deliberately hide the truth of what they have seen. This is the sole reason for the countless theories relating to the Theory of Evolution. The moment they accept the existence and majesty of Allah, they are obliged to submit to His will, which is an extremely difficult proposition for arrogant people. The Qur'an again sheds light on the plight of such people who take up a stance of an ignorant arrogance against Allah:

They repudiated them wrongly and haughtily, in spite of their own certainty about them.... (Surat an-Naml: 14)

There are those who, for the sake of denying the existence of Allah, struggle to uphold the falsehood of evolution with a variety of theories that are far from any scientific or logical basis. Such is their determination that they defend their views with extremely ridiculous examples, claiming that such a sophisticated and complex system such as the immune system has developed in stages from a single antibody.

Those scientists who have become aware of the situation they are in have started to distance themselves from evolutionary associations, realizing the shameful nature of such explanations.

Another group of scientists accept the theory of evolution, not because it is accurate and they believe in it, but because there is no other theory to support their denial of Allah's existence.

However, there is no obligation to accept and follow a certain theory. When people become curious about the creation of the universe and its contents, it will be sufficient for them to assess the self-evident truths objectively and with a free mind.

As we have continuously stressed in this book, there is not a shred of evidence based on any trials, experiments or observations that could support the claims of the theory of evolution. Scientific disciplines such as biology, biochemistry, microbiology, genetics, palaeontology and anatomy have made it clear that the theory of evolution is an imaginary hypothesis about events which have never taken place and nor can ever take place. (See the chapter on "The Evolution Deceit").

Today, all research carried out in various branches of science, shows that all living and non-living beings on the earth and in the sky have been created by an all-powerful and almighty Creator Who possesses eternal wisdom, knowledge and might. To see this fact, and to understand the fictitious nature of fabricated theories, such as that of evolution, advanced technology or scientific knowledge is not necessarily required. Allah has displayed the evidence of His existence and creation for everyone who has a clear mind and conscience to see, irrespective of which historical era he lives in, be it the dark ages or the middle ages:

> **In the creation of the heavens and earth, and the alternation of the night and day, and the ships which sail the seas to people's benefit, and the water which Allah sends down from the sky – by which He brings the earth to life when it was dead and scatters about on it creatures of every kind – and the varying direction of the winds, and the clouds subservient between heaven and earth, there are Signs for people who use their intellect. (Surat al-Baqara: 164)**

The duty that falls to those people of understanding, who can grasp the above verse fully, is to constantly recall the obvious "fact of creation" evident in the whole universe from the cells to giant galaxies, by quoting the following words of the Qur'an;

> **…Your Lord is the Lord of the heavens and the earth, He who brought them into being. I am one of those who bear witness to that. (Surat al-Anbiya: 56)**

THE EVOLUTION DECEIT

Every detail in this universe points to a superior creation. By contrast, materialism, which seeks to deny the fact of creation in the universe, is nothing but an unscientific fallacy.

Once materialism is invalidated, all other theories based on this philosophy are rendered baseless. Foremost of them is Darwinism, that is, the theory of evolution. This theory, which argues that life originated from inanimate matter through coincidences, has been demolished with the recognition that the universe was created by Allah. American astrophysicist Hugh Ross explains this as follows:

> Atheism, Darwinism, and virtually all the "isms" emanating from the eighteenth to the twentieth century philosophies are built upon the assumption, the incorrect assumption, that the universe is infinite. The singularity has brought us face to face with the cause – or causer – beyond/behind/before the universe and all that it contains, including life itself. [19]

It is Allah Who created the universe and Who designed it down to its smallest detail. Therefore, it is impossible for the theory of evolution, which holds that living beings are not created by Allah, but are products of coincidences, to be true.

Unsurprisingly, when we look at the theory of evolution, we see that this theory is denounced by scientific findings. The design in life is extremely complex and striking. In the inanimate world, for instance, we can explore how sensitive are the balances which atoms rest upon, and further, in the animate world, we can observe in what complex designs these atoms were brought together, and how extraordinary are the mechanisms and structures such as proteins, enzymes, and cells, which are manufactured with them.

This extraordinary design in life invalidated Darwinism at the end of the 20th century.

We have dealt with this subject in great detail in some of our other studies, and shall continue to do so. However, we think that, considering its importance, it will be helpful to make a short summary here as well.

The Scientific Collapse of Darwinism

Although a doctrine going back as far as ancient Greece, the theory of evolution was advanced extensively in the 19th century. The most important development that made the theory the top topic of the world of science was the book by Charles Darwin titled *"The Origin of Species"* published in 1859. In this book, Darwin denied that different living species on the earth were created separately by Allah. According to Darwin, all living beings had a common ancestor and they diversified over time through small changes.

Darwin's theory was not based on any concrete scientific finding; as he also accepted, it was just an "assumption." Moreover, as Darwin confessed in the long chapter of his book titled "Difficulties of the Theory," the theory was failing in the face of many critical questions.

Darwin invested all his hopes in new scientific discoveries, which he expected to solve the "Difficulties of the Theory." However, contrary to his expectations, scientific findings expanded the dimensions of these difficulties.

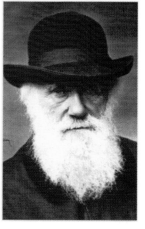

Charles Darwin

The defeat of Darwinism against science can be reviewed under three basic topics:

1) The theory can by no means explain how life originated on the earth.

2) There is no scientific finding showing that the "evolutionary mechanisms" proposed by the theory have any power to evolve at all.

3) The fossil record proves completely the contrary of the suggestions of the theory of evolution.

In this section, we will examine these three basic points in general outlines:

The First Insurmountable Step:
The Origin of Life

The theory of evolution posits that all living species evolved from a single living cell that emerged on the primitive earth 3.8 billion years ago. How a single cell could generate millions of complex living species and, if such an evolution really occurred, why traces of it cannot be observed in the fossil record are some of the questions the theory cannot answer. However, first and foremost, of the first step of the alleged evolutionary process it has to be inquired: How did this "first cell" originate?

Since the theory of evolution denies creation and does not accept any kind of supernatural intervention, it maintains that the "first cell" originated coincidentally within the laws of nature, without any design, plan, or arrangement. According to the theory, inanimate matter must have produced a living cell as a result of coincidences. This, however, is a claim inconsistent with even the most unassailable rules of biology.

"Life Comes from Life"

In his book, Darwin never referred to the origin of life. The primitive understanding of science in his time rested on the assumption that living beings had a very simple structure. Since medieval times, spontaneous generation, the theory asserting that non-living materials came together to form living organisms, had been widely accepted. It was commonly believed that insects came into being from food leftovers, and mice from wheat. Interesting experiments were conducted to prove this theory. Some wheat was placed on a dirty piece of cloth, and it was believed that mice would originate from it after a while.

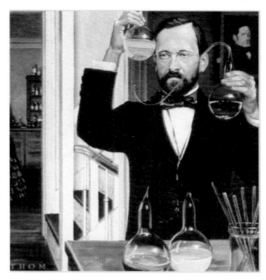

Louis Pasteur invalidated the claim that "inanimate matter can create life", which constituted the groundwork of the theory of evolution, with the experiments he carried out.

Similarly, worms developing in meat was assumed to be evidence of spontaneous generation. However, only some time later was it understood that worms did not appear on meat spontaneously, but were carried there by flies in the form of larvae, invisible to the naked eye.

Even in the period when Darwin wrote *The Origin of Species*, the belief that bacteria could come into existence from non-living matter was widely accepted in the world of science.

However, five years after Darwin's book was published, the discovery of Louis Pasteur disproved this belief, which constituted the groundwork of evolution. Pasteur summarized the conclusion he reached after time-consuming studies and experiments: *"The claim that inanimate matter can originate life is buried in history for good."* [20]

Advocates of the theory of evolution resisted the findings of Pasteur for a long time. However, as the development of science unraveled the complex structure of the cell of a living being, the idea that life could come into being coincidentally faced an even greater impasse.

Inconclusive Efforts in the 20th Century

The first evolutionist who took up the subject of the origin of life in the 20th century was the renowned Russian biologist Alexander Oparin. With various theses he advanced in the 1930's, he tried to prove that the cell of a living being could originate by coincidence. These studies, however, were doomed to failure, and Oparin had to make the following confession: "Unfortunately, the origin of the cell remains a question which is actually the darkest point of the entire evolution theory." [21]

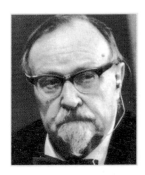

Alexander Oparin's attempts to bring an evolutionist explanation to the origin of life ended in a great fiasco.

Evolutionist followers of Oparin tried to carry out experiments to solve the problem of the origin of life. The best known of these experiments was carried out by American chemist Stanley Miller in 1953. Combining the gases he alleged to have existed in the primordial earth's atmosphere in an experiment set-up, and adding energy to the mixture, Miller synthesized several organic molecules (amino acids) present in the structure of proteins.

Barely a few years had passed before it was revealed that this experiment, which was then presented as an important step in the name of evolution, was invalid, the atmosphere used in the experiment having been very different from real earth conditions. [22]

After a long silence, Miller confessed that the atmosphere medium he used was unrealistic. [23]

All the evolutionist efforts put forth throughout the 20th century to explain the origin of life ended with failure. The geochemist Jeffrey Bada from San Diego Scripps Institute accepts this fact in an article published in *Earth* Magazine in 1998:

Today as we leave the twentieth century, we still face the biggest unsolved problem that we had when we entered the twentieth century: How did life originate on Earth? [24]

The Complex Structure of Life

The primary reason why the theory of evolution ended up in such a big impasse about the origin of life is that even the living organisms deemed the simplest have incredibly complex structures. The cell of a living being is more complex than all of the technological products produced by man. Today, even in the most developed laboratories of the world, a living cell cannot be produced by bringing inorganic materials together.

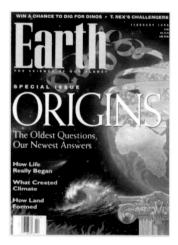

As accepted also by the latest evolutionist sources, the origin of life is still a great stumbling block for the theory of evolution.

The conditions required for the formation of a cell are too great in quantity to be explained away by coincidences. The probability of proteins, the building blocks of cell, being synthesized coincidentally, is 1 in 10^{950} for an average protein made up of 500 amino acids. In mathematics, a probability smaller than 1 over 10^{50} is practically considered to be impossible.

The DNA molecule, which is located in the nucleus of the cell and which stores genetic information, is an incredible databank. It is calculated that if the information coded in DNA were written down, this would make a giant library consisting of 900 volumes of encyclopaedias of 500 pages each.

A very interesting dilemma emerges at this point: the DNA can only replicate with the help of some specialized proteins (enzymes). However, the synthesis of these enzymes can only be realized by the information coded in DNA. As they both depend on each other, they have to exist at the same time for replication. This brings the scenario that life originated by itself to a deadlock. Prof. Leslie Orgel, an evolutionist of repute from the University of San Diego, California, confesses this fact in the September 1994 issue of the *Scientific American* magazine:

It is extremely improbable that proteins and nucleic acids, both of which are structurally complex, arose spontaneously in the same place at the same time. Yet it also seems impossible to have one without the other. And so, at first glance, one might have to conclude that life could never, in fact, have originated by chemical means. [25]

No doubt, if it is impossible for life to have originated from natural causes, then it has to be accepted that life was "created" in a supernatural way. This fact explicitly invalidates the theory of evolution, whose main purpose is to deny creation.

Imaginary Mechanisms of Evolution

The second important point that negates Darwin's theory is that both concepts put forward by the theory as "evolutionary mechanisms" were understood to have, in reality, no evolutionary power.

Darwin based his evolution allegation entirely on the mechanism of "natural selection". The importance he placed on this mechanism was evident in the name of his book: *The Origin of Species, By Means Of Natural Selection...*

Natural selection holds that those living things that are stronger and more suited to the natural conditions of their habitats will survive in the struggle for life. For example, in a deer herd under the threat of attack by wild animals, those that can run faster will survive. Therefore, the deer herd will be comprised of faster and stronger individuals. However, unquestionably, this mechanism will not cause deer to evolve and transform themselves into another living species, for instance, horses.

Therefore, the mechanism of natural selection has no evolutionary power. Darwin was also aware of this fact and had to state this in his book *"The Origin of Species:"*

Natural selection can do nothing until favourable variations chance to occur.[26]

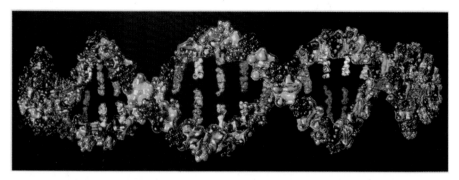

One of the facts nullifying the theory of evolution is the incredibly complex structure of life. DNA molecule located in the nucleus of cells of living beings is an example of this. DNA is a sort of databank formed of the arrangement of four different molecules in different sequences. This databank contains the codes of all the physical traits of a living being. When the human DNA is put into writing, it is calculated that this would result in an encyclopaedia made up of 900 volumes. Unquestionably, such extraordinary information definitely refutes the concept of coincidence.

Lamarck's Impact

So, how could these "favourable variations" occur? Darwin tried to answer this question from the standpoint of the primitive understanding of science in his age. According to the French biologist Lamarck, who lived before Darwin, living creatures passed on the traits they acquired during their lifetime to the next generation and these traits, accumulating from one generation to another, caused new species to be formed. For instance, according to Lamarck, giraffes evolved from antelopes; as they struggled to eat the leaves of high trees, their necks were extended from generation to generation.

Darwin also gave similar examples, and in his book *"The Origin of Species,"* for instance, said that some bears going into water to find food transformed themselves into whales over time. [27]

However, the laws of inheritance discovered by Mendel and verified by the science of genetics that flourished in the 20th century, utterly demolished the legend that acquired traits were passed on to subsequent generations. Thus, natural selection fell out of favour as an evolutionary mechanism.

Neo-Darwinism and Mutations

In order to find a solution, Darwinists advanced the "Modern Synthetic Theory", or as it is more commonly known, Neo-Darwinism, at the end of the 1930's. Neo-Darwinism added mutations, which are distortions formed in the genes of living beings because of external factors such as radiation or replication errors, as the "cause of favourable variations" in addition to natural mutation.

Today, the model that stands for evolution in the world is Neo-Darwinism. The theory maintains that millions of living beings present on the earth formed as a result of a process whereby numerous complex organs of these organisms such as the ears, eyes, lungs, and wings, underwent "mutations," that is, genetic disorders. Yet, there is an outright scientific fact that totally undermines this theory: Mutations do not cause living beings to develop; on the contrary, they always cause harm to them.

The reason for this is very simple: the DNA has a very complex structure and random effects can only cause harm to it. American geneticist B.G. Ranganathan explains this as follows:

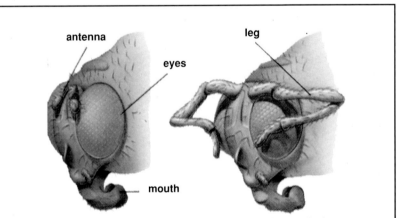

antenna   leg

eyes

mouth

Since the beginning of the century, evolutionists have tried to produce mutations in fruit flies, and offer this as an example of useful mutation. However, the only result obtained at the end of these efforts that lasted for decades were disfigured, diseased and defective flies. Above is the head of a normal fruit fly and on the right is the head of a mutated fruit fly.

Mutations are small, random, and harmful. They rarely occur and the best possibility is that they will be ineffectual. These four characteristics of mutations imply that mutations cannot lead to an evolutionary development. A random change in a highly specialised organism is either ineffectual or harmful. A random change in a watch cannot improve the watch. It will most probably harm it or at best be ineffectual. An earthquake does not improve the city, it brings destruction. [28]

Not surprisingly, no mutation example, which is useful, that is, which is observed to develop the genetic code, has been observed so far. All mutations have proved to be harmful. It was understood that mutation, which is presented as an "evolutionary mechanism," is actually a genetic occurrence that harms living beings, and leaves them disabled. (The

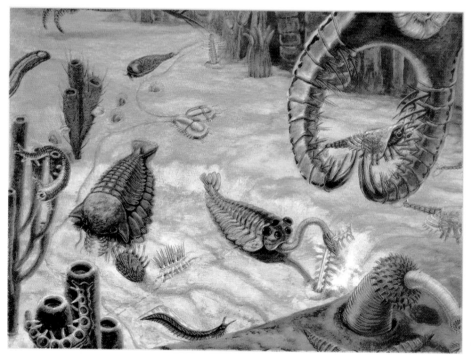

The theory of evolution claims that living species gradually evolved from one another. The fossil record, however, explicitly falsifies this claim. For example, in the Cambrian Period, some 550 million years ago, dozens of totally distinct living species suddenly emerged. These living beings depicted in the above picture have very complex structures. This fact, referred to as the "Cambrian Explosion" in scientific literature, is plain evidence of creation.

most common effect of mutation on human beings is cancer). No doubt, a destructive mechanism cannot be an "evolutionary mechanism." Natural selection, on the other hand, "can do nothing by itself" as Darwin also accepted. This fact shows us that there is no "evolutionary mechanism" in nature. Since no evolutionary mechanism exists, neither could any imaginary process called evolution have taken place.

The Fossil Record: No Sign of Intermediate Forms

The clearest evidence that the scenario suggested by the theory of evolution did not take place is the fossil record.

According to the theory of evolution, every living species has sprung from a predecessor. A previously existing species turned into something else in time and all species have come into being in this way. According to the theory, this transformation proceeds gradually over millions of years.

Had this been the case, then numerous intermediary species should have existed and lived within this long transformation period.

For instance, some half-fish/half-reptiles should have lived in the past which had acquired some reptilian traits in addition to the fish traits they already had. Or there should have existed some reptile-birds, which acquired some bird traits in addition to the reptilian traits they already had. Since these would be in a transitional phase, they should be disabled, defective, crippled living beings. Evolutionists refer to these imaginary creatures, which they believe to have lived in the past, as "transitional forms."

If such animals had really existed, there should be millions and even billions of them in number and variety. More importantly, the remains of these strange creatures should be present in the fossil record. In *The Origin of Species*, Darwin explained:

> *If my theory be true, numberless intermediate varieties, linking most closely all of the species of the same group together must assuredly have existed... Consequently, evidence of their former existence could be found only amongst fossil remains.*[29]

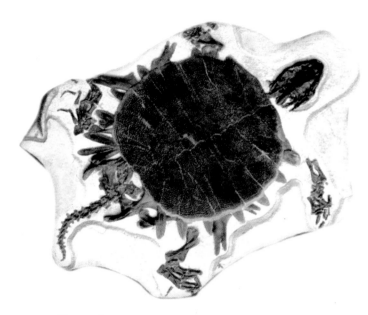

The fossil record rises like a great barricade in front of the theory of evolution, for it shows that living species emerged suddenly and fully-formed, without any evolutionary transitional forms between them. This fact is evidence that species are separately created.

Darwin's Hopes Shattered

However, although evolutionists have been making strenuous efforts to find fossils since the middle of the 19th century all over the world, no transitional forms have yet been uncovered. All the fossils unearthed in excavations showed that, contrary to the expectations of evolutionists, life appeared on earth all of a sudden and fully-formed.

A famous British paleontologist, Derek V. Ager, admits this fact, even though he is an evolutionist:

> *The point emerges that if we examine the fossil rec,ord in detail, whether at the level of orders or of species, we find — over and over again — not gradual evolution, but the sudden explosion of one group at the expense of another.*[30]

This means that in the fossil record, all living species suddenly emerge as fully formed, without any intermediate forms in between. This is just the opposite of Darwin's assumptions. Also, it is very strong evidence that living beings are created. The only explanation of a living species emerging suddenly and complete in every detail without any evolutionary ancestor can be that this species was created. This fact is admitted also by the widely known evolutionist biologist Douglas Futuyma:

Creation and evolution, between them, exhaust the possible explanations for the origin of living things. Organisms either appeared on the earth fully developed or they did not. If they did not, they must have developed from pre-existing species by some process of modification. If they did appear in a fully developed state, they must indeed have been created by some omnipotent intelligence. [31]

Fossils show that living beings emerged fully developed and in a perfect state on the earth. That means that "the origin of species" is, contrary to Darwin's supposition, not evolution but creation.

The Tale of Human Evolution

The subject most often brought up by the advocates of the theory of evolution is the subject of the origin of man. The Darwinist claim holds that the modern men of today evolved from some kind of ape-like creatures. During this alleged evolutionary process, which is supposed to have started 4-5 million years ago, it is claimed that there existed some "transitional forms" between modern man and his ancestors. According to this completely imaginary scenario, four basic "categories" are listed:

1. Australopithecus
2. Homo habilis
3. Homo erectus
4. Homo sapiens

Evolutionists call the so-called first ape-like ancestors of men "Australopithecus" which means "South African ape." These living beings are actually nothing but an old ape species that has become extinct. Extensive research done on various Australopithecus specimens by two world famous anatomists from England and the USA, namely, Lord Solly Zuckerman and Prof. Charles Oxnard, has shown that these belonged to an ordinary ape species that became extinct and bore no resemblance to humans.[32]

Evolutionists classify the next stage of human evolution as "homo," that is "man." According to the evolutionist claim, the living beings in the Homo series are more developed than Australopithecus. Evolutionists devise a fanciful evolution scheme by arranging different fossils of these creatures in a particular order. This scheme is imaginary because it has never been proved that there is an evolutionary relation between these different classes. Ernst Mayr, one of the foremost defenders of the theory of evolution in the 20th century, admits this fact by saying that "the chain reaching as far as Homo sapiens is actually lost." [33]

By outlining the link chain as "Australopithecus > Homo habilis > Homo erectus > Homo sapiens," evolutionists imply that each of these species is one another's ancestor. However, recent findings of paleoanthropologists have revealed that Australopithecus, Homo habilis and Homo erectus lived at different parts of the world at the same time.[34]

Moreover, a certain segment of humans classified as Homo erectus have lived up until very modern times. Homo sapiens neandarthalensis and Homo sapiens sapiens (modern man) co-existed in the same region.[35]

This situation apparently indicates the invalidity of the claim that they are ancestors of one another. A paleontologist from Harvard University, Stephen Jay Gould, explains this deadlock of the theory of evolution although he is an evolutionist himself:

> *What has become of our ladder if there are three coexisting lineages of hominids (A. africanus, the robust australopithecines, and H. habilis), none clearly derived from another? Moreover, none of the three display any evolutionary trends during their tenure on earth.* [36]

Put briefly, the scenario of human evolution, which is sought to be upheld with the help of various drawings of some "half ape, half human" creatures appearing in the media and course books, that is, frankly, by means of propaganda, is nothing but a tale with no scientific ground.

Lord Solly Zuckerman, one of the most famous and respected scientists in the U.K., who carried out research on this subject for years, and particularly studied Australopithecus fossils for 15 years, finally concluded, despite being an evolutionist himself, that there is, in fact, no such family tree branching out from ape-like creatures to man.

Zuckerman also made an interesting "spectrum of science." He formed a spectrum of sciences ranging from those he considered scientific to those he considered unscientific. According to Zuckerman's spectrum, the most "scientific"–that is, depending on concrete data–fields of science are chemistry and physics. After them come the biological sciences and then the social sciences. At the far end of the spectrum, which is the part considered to be most "unscientific," are "extra-sensory perception"–concepts such as telepathy and sixth sense–and finally "human evolution." Zuckerman explains his reasoning:

> We then move right off the register of objective truth into those fields of presumed biological science, like extrasensory perception or the interpretation of man's fossil history, where to the faithful (evolutionist) anything is possible - and where the ardent believer (in evolution) is sometimes able to believe several contradictory things at the same time. [37]

The tale of human evolution boils down to nothing but the prejudiced interpretations of some fossils unearthed by certain people, who blindly adhere to their theory.

A Materialist Faith

The information we have presented so far shows us that the theory of evolution is a claim evidently at variance with scientific findings. The theory's claim on the origin of life is inconsistent with science, the evolutionary mechanisms it proposes have no evolutionary power, and fossils demonstrate that the intermediate forms required by the theory never existed. So, it certainly follows that the theory of evolution should be pushed aside as an unscientific idea. This is how many ideas such as the earth-centered universe model have been taken out of the agenda of science throughout history.

However, the theory of evolution is pressingly kept on the agenda of science. Some people even try to represent criticisms directed against the theory as an "attack on science." Why?

The reason is that the theory of evolution is an indispensable dog-matic belief for some circles. These circles are blindly devoted to materi-alist philosophy and adopt Darwinism because it is the only materialist explanation that can be put forward for the workings of nature.

Interestingly enough, they also confess this fact from time to time. A well known geneticist and an outspoken evolutionist, Richard C. Lewon-tin from Harvard University, confesses that he is "first and foremost a ma-terialist and then a scientist":

> *It is not that the methods and institutions of science somehow compel us ac-cept a material explanation of the phenomenal world, but, on the contrary, that we are forced by our a priori adherence to material causes to create an apparatus of investigation and a set of concepts that produce material expla-nations, no matter how counter-intuitive, no matter how mystifying to the uninitiated. Moreover, that materialism is absolute, so we cannot allow a Divine Foot in the door.* [38]

These are explicit statements that Darwinism is a dogma kept alive just for the sake of adherence to the materialist philosophy. This dogma maintains that there is no being save matter. Therefore, it argues that in-animate, unconscious matter created life. It insists that millions of differ-ent living species; for instance, birds, fish, giraffes, tigers, insects, trees, flowers, whales and human beings originated as a result of the interac-tions between matter such as the pouring rain, the lightning flash, etc., out of inanimate matter. This is a precept contrary both to reason and science. Yet Darwinists continue to defend it just so as "not to allow a Divine Foot in the door."

Anyone who does not look at the origin of living beings with a ma-terialist prejudice will see this evident truth: All living beings are works of a Creator, Who is All-Powerful, All-Wise and All-Knowing. This Crea-tor is Allah, Who created the whole universe from non-existence, de-signed it in the most perfect form, and fashioned all living beings.

They said 'Glory be to You!
We have no knowledge except what You have taught us.
You are the All-Knowing, the All-Wise.'
(Surat al-Baqarah: 32)

NOTES

1. Edward Edelson *The Immune System, Chelsea House Publisher, 1989, p. 13-14*
2. George Gamow, *One Two Three... Infinity*, Bantam Books, 1971, p. 245
3. Ali Demirsoy, *Kalıtım ve Evrim* (Inheritance and Evolution), Ankara: Meteksan Yayınları p. 416
4. *Scientific American,* September 1993, p. 54
5. Ali Demirsoy, *Kalıtım ve Evrim* (Inheritance and Evolution), Ankara: Meteksan Yayınları p. 61
6. *Scientific American,* September 1993, p. 65
7. Ali Demirsoy, *Kalıtım ve Evrim* (Inheritance and Evolution), Ankara: Meteksan Yayınları p. 79
8. Michael J. Behe, *Darwin's Black Box,* New York: Free Press, 1996, p. 30
9. *Scientific American,* September 1993, p. 58
10. Mahlon B. Hoagland, *Roots Of Life,* p. 106-107
11. *Bilim ve Teknik Dergisi* (Journal of Science and Technology), Vol 26, No 309, August 1993 p. 567
12. Michael J. Behe, *Darwin's Black Box,* New York: Free Press, 1996, p. 39
13. Charles Darwin, *The Origin of Species: A Facsimile of the First Edition,* Harvard University Press, 1964, p. 204
14. Stephen Jay Gould, *"Not Necessarily a Wing",* Natural History, October 1985, p. 13
15. J. A. Endler ve T. McLellan (1988), "The Process of Evolution: Toward A Newer Synthesis", *Annual Review of Ecology and Systematics,* 19, 397
16. Pierre P. Grassé, *Evolution of Living Organisms,* New York, 1977, p. 88s
17. Klaus Dose (1988), "The Origin Of Life: More Questions Than Answers", *Interdisciplinary Science Reviews,* 13, 348
18. Francis Darwin, *Life and Letters of Charles Darwin,* Charles Darwin to W.B. Carpenter
19. Hugh Ross, *The Fingerprint of God,* p. 50
20. Sidney Fox, Klaus Dose, *Molecular Evolution and The Origin of Life,* New York: Marcel Dekker, 1977. p. 2
21. Alexander I. Oparin, *Origin of Life,* (1936) New York, Dover Publications, 1953 (Reprint), p.196
22. "New Evidence on Evolution of Early Atmosphere and Life", *Bulletin of the American Meteorological Society,* vol. 63, November 1982, p. 1328-1330.
23. Stanley Miller, *Molecular Evolution of Life: Current Status of the Prebiotic Synthesis of Small Molecules,* 1986, p. 7
24. Jeffrey Bada, *Earth,* February 1998, p. 40
25. Leslie E. Orgel, *"The Origin of Life on Earth",* Scientific American, Vol 271, October 1994, p. 78
26. Charles Darwin, *The Origin of Species: A Facsimile of the First Edition,* Harvard University Press, 1964, p. 189
27. Charles Darwin, *The Origin of Species: A Facsimile of the First Edition,* Harvard University Press, 1964, p. 184.
28. B. G. Ranganathan, *Origins?,* Pennsylvania: The Banner Of Truth Trust, 1988.
29. Charles Darwin, *The Origin of Species: A Facsimile of the First Edition,* Harvard University Press, 1964, p. 179
30. Derek A. Ager, *"The Nature of the Fossil Record",* Proceedings of the British Geological Association, vol. 87, 1976, p. 133
31. Douglas J. Futuyma, *Science on Trial,* New York: Pantheon Books, 1983. p. 197
32. Solly Zuckerman, *Beyond The Ivory Tower,* New York: Toplinger Publications, 1970, ss. 75-94; Charles E. Oxnard, *"The Place of Australopithecines in Human Evolution: Grounds for Doubt",* Nature, Vol. 258, p. 389
33. J. Rennie, *"Darwin's Current Bulldog: Ernst Mayr",* Scientific American, December 1992
34. Alan Walker, Science, vol. 207, 1980, p. 1103; A. J. Kelso, Physical Antropology, 1st ed., New York: J. B. Lipincott Co., 1970, p. 221; M. D. Leakey, Olduvai Gorge, vol. 3, Cambridge: Cambridge University Press, 1971, p. 272
35. Time, November 1996
36. S. J. Gould, *Natural History,* vol. 85, 1976, p. 30
37. Solly Zuckerman, *Beyond The Ivory Tower,* New York: Toplinger Publications, 1970, p. 19
38. Richard Lewontin, *"The Demon-Haunted World",* The New York Review of Books, 9 January, 1997, p. 28